Swanson

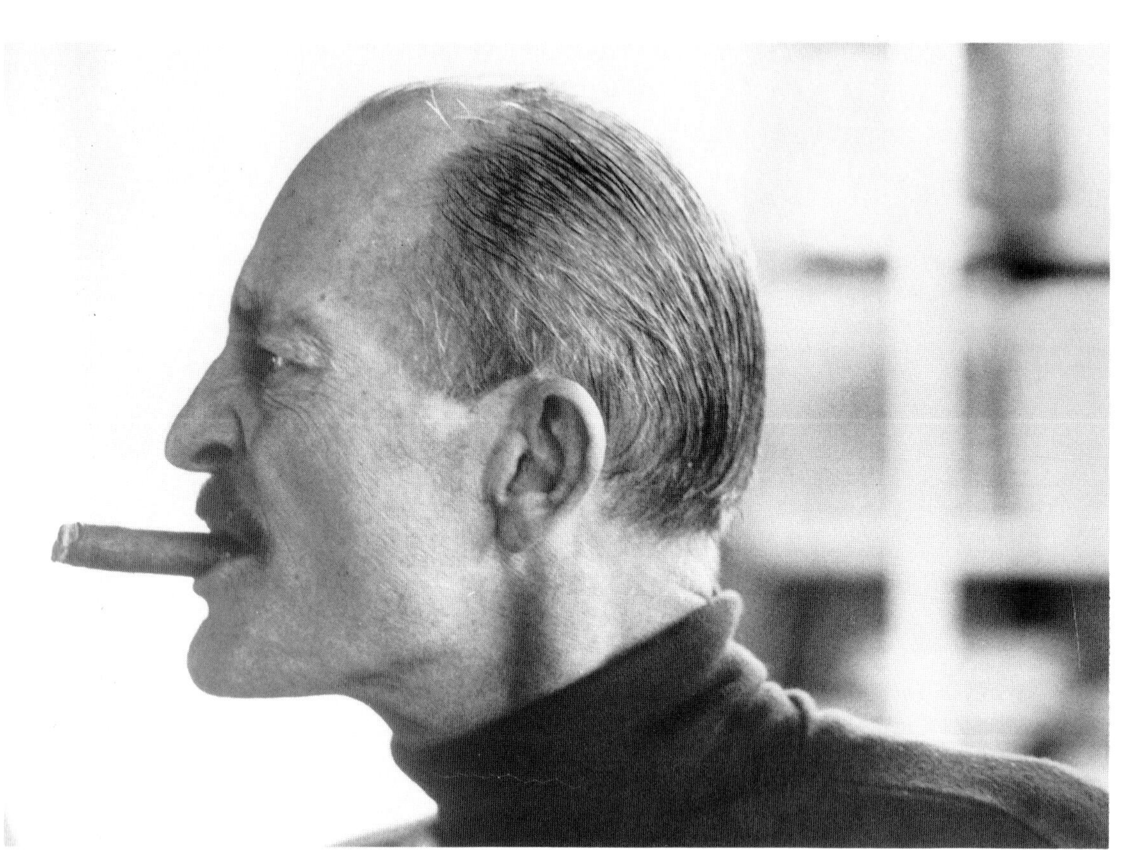

LETTERS FROM H.C. WESTERMANN

Selected and edited by Bill Barrette
Biographical Sketch by Joanna Beall Westermann

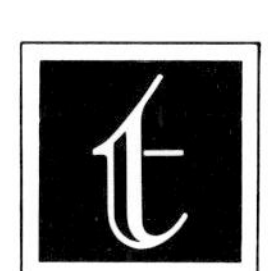

TIMKEN PUBLISHERS, INC.
New York

Printed and bound in The United States of America

ISBN 0-943221-00-5

Library of Congress Cataloging-in-Publication Data

Westermann, H.C. (Horace Clifford), 1922-
Letters from H.C. Westermann.

1. Westermann, H.C. (Horace Clifford), 1922- —Correspondence. 2. Sculptors—United States—Correspondence. 3. Drawing, American. 4. Drawing, 20th century—United States. 5. Artists' preparatory studies—United States. I. Barrette, Bill. II. Westermann, Joanna Beall. III. Title. NB237.W44A3 1988 709'.2'4 [B] 87-17985 ISBN 0-943221-00-5

Frontispiece: H. C. Westermann, August 1981. Photo, Bobbe Wolf.

Contents

PREFACE

The letters here represent only a selection of H.C. Westermann's large correspondence. They are arranged in separate chapters and follow the themes given in the chapter headings. Within these chapters they are arranged chronologically. A list of all the letters reproduced can be found at the end of the book. Westermann sent these letters in extraordinary illustrated envelopes only one of which we are able to include here.

Westermann's handwritten unillustrated letters have been transcribed into type. Minor corrections of spelling and grammar have been made to aid legibility. We have reproduced more than fifty of the illustrated letters in color. Of the remaining illustrated letters, most of them are pen and ink drawings. Measurements of the letters are given in inches with height preceding width. Photographs on pages 137, 140, 141 and 144 are from the collection of Bill Barrette. All other photographs are from the collection of Joanna Beall Westermann.

Many people have cooperated to make this book possible. In particular, Joanna Beall Westermann has offered constant assistance. She has given us names of people to contact for letters and, in a number of cases, she has contacted them herself. She has provided the watercolor of wood grain that is on the cover and finally she has written the biographical sketch that gives us an overview of Westermann's life which is at once personal and reliable. Allan and Jean Frumkin have been very generous allowing repeated visits to their house to both study and photograph Westermann's letters. It was after seeing their very large collection of Westermann's letters that we realized the letters would make a worthwhile book. More than fifty people have sent us slides, xeroxes and, in a number of cases, the letters themselves. Their willing cooperation is a remarkable testimony to the special regard which they had for Westermann. We would like to thank Martha Renner, Dennis Adrian, Edwin Janss, Billy Al Bengston, Terry and Jo Harvey Allen, Noma Copley, William Copley, Billy Copley, Bruce and Doris Oxford, Betty Asher, Gerald W. Bush, Jim Corcoran, William Wiley, Ed Ruscha, Xavier Fourcade, Peter Freeman, Barbara Haskell, Mike Nevelson, Gene Bowen, Roger Brouard, Ellen Lanyon, Tom Armstrong and the staff of the Whitney Museum, Herk van Tongeren, Ken Price, Richard Riesman, Jerry Ordover, Robert and Rhett Delford Brown, Robert and Mavis Hudson, Al Shean, Cheryl Flood, Gilbert H. Kinney, Richard Hollander and the Spencer Museum of Art. We would also like to thank a number of other people who have been involved in this project: Linda Norden and Robert Storr for their editorial advice, Louise Fili for her cover design, Lynton Gardiner for photographing the bulk of these letters, Annabel Levitt for her book design and editorial assistance, and finally Fred Kleeberg for so ably overseeing the production of this book from its beginning.

— Jane Timken, *Publisher* and Bill Barrette, *Editor*

INTRODUCTION

This is a book of letters and of drawings sent as letters. It is only part of an enormous correspondence that the sculptor H.C. Westermann (1922-1981) conducted with hundreds of sympathetic souls with whom he wished to share his idiosyncratic view of the world. We will never know how many letters exist, for with the exception of a letter to his doctor in 1976, he never made any copies. It is rare in this era of the telephone to have such a large and consistent correspondence and even more rare to have one that is so heavily illustrated. Why did Westermann send so many letters? A great many of them are ostensibly thank you notes or replies to letters, and the impression on glancing through them is one of an almost exaggerated sincerity and politeness, albeit presented in a colorful package. But a casual glimpse shows that the letters were far more than simple communication. His wife Joanna Beall Westermann has said that the letter writing, or perhaps more accurately letter drawing, served to release the extreme tension he felt working on his pieces, and that he habitually spent a couple of hours every morning writing and drawing. The letters are written directly from the heart and as such they provide us with a unique kind of drawn autobiography with captions. These letters have for the most part never been seen before, so in a sense they stand as a new body of work by this artist and equally they contain information which helps us understand his sculpture.

Before talking of the letters we should first consider his career and character as an artist. For more than twenty years H.C. Westermann has been well known in the art world as the creator of a deeply felt and often disturbing body of sculpture. But because of the fierce individualism of his vision, his insistence on originality and indifference to trends, it has been difficult to place his work within the rapid succession of styles that followed the wake of Abstract Expressionism. Westermann certainly plays a significant role in the development of the West Coast "Funk" and Chicago Imagist schools as well as much that is happening now. In 1978 his importance as a major post-war sculptor was acknowledged by the Whitney Museum with a large-scale retrospective and traveling exhibition. Still, despite general recognition and wide-ranging influence, Westermann's work remains highly esteemed but poorly understood.

The artist with whom Westermann has been most often compared is Joseph Cornell, primarily because both made enigmatic boxes. Their differences as these letters make clear are, however, far greater than their apparent similarities. Westermann was insistently American in his outlook, expressing disdain for things foreign. The references in his sculpture are never random, but are always directly based on deeply personal experience. While nostalgia plays an important role in both artists' work, Cornell's is that of a romanticized reverie, while Westermann's is rather a melancholy longing for home, for a native place. His mother's death from tuberculosis when he was nineteen, his father's remarriage, and Westermann's separation from his family and his experience during World War II all contributed to his conviction that the world was no longer a safe and nourishing place. Westermann was affected by these events to an unusual degree and concluded that the individual was powerless to control ever-present forces of destruction. In a letter to his sister Martha upon visiting his childhood home he wrote of this sense of alienation, "I went back to Norwich Drive and you know there's just nothing there anymore — I mean like where our home used to be. It was like we had never had a home or a family or even been born — none of us."

This sense of loss and the insecurity based on never again finding a safe haven also explain the emphasis Westermann placed on the details and finish of his sculptures and accounts for the extravagant care he lavished on the house and studio he was to build in Connecticut. It is this insistence on "rightness" that has led critics to inevitably mention Westermann's connection with craft. But Westermann disliked the idea of craft per se. Rather the perfection he demonstrated toward the execution of his sculpture served a more specifically psychic need. His heightened sense of vulnerability and concern for the fate of his pieces led him to make them as strong as possible so as to insure their chances of survival in an indifferent or possibly hostile environment once they were released from his care. His work might more profitably be thought of as containers for strong and often ambiguous statements that depend on the alertness and ingenuity of the viewer for full comprehension, not as a highly crafted variety of the surrealist box.

It is important to be aware of Westermann's education as well as his early success because he has often been mistaken for some kind of American primitive. After serving in two wars with a brief stint as an acrobat in the United Service Organization in between, Westermann returned to Chicago to take a degree in fine arts at the Chicago Art Institute. He had previously studied advertising and design there in the later 1940s. After graduating from the Art Institute he began making his singular constructions and soon received recognition. Allan Frumkin became his dealer in 1956. And in 1959 he was included in the New Images of Man exhibition at the Museum of Modern Art. The titles of his sculptures and the references in his letters as well as his education demonstrate that he was completely familiar with the canons of modernism, even as he chose to speak with his own particular voice. As a student he was particularly attracted to the work of Paul Klee which he saw at the Arts Club of Chicago. And before he abandoned painting for sculpture in 1954, his work shows the influence of Klee more than any other artist. He also admired the work of Duchamp and Brancusi. His *Lop Lop* letter is a direct reference to Max Ernst, taken from *La Femme de cent têtes*. One of his pieces from 1965 is dedicated to Elie Nadelman. At the same time he was very much attracted to a more unorthodox tradition. He often expressed his admiration for "real" artists amongst whom he included his maternal uncle and maternal grandfather, as well as a number of anonymous artists, even a string collector who created a ball of string so large that it filled an entire room in his house.

In fact Westermann's outlook was a distinctly American one and in particular reflected the experience of growing up in California in the thirties and participating both in World War II and in the Korean War. He was a gunner on the USS Enterprise during the Second World War and saw numerous kamikaze attacks. He would refer to these episodes again and again, first in drawings and then in sculpture beginning in 1965. And finally as if the drawings and sculpture were not enough, he began somewhat apologetically to write about the experience. Westermann stands apart from other visual artists of the post-war period in the way that his work is able to integrate images of his experiences in such a direct manner. This sensibility was in some respects closer to the writers of his generation. He writes on one of these Death Ship letters, "Here is the same drawing I love to do. Hundreds by now. This drawing is like learning a handstand. They vary of course. I never get tired of it and maybe someday I'll learn how." And in another letter, this time a drawing for a sculpture *Death Ship Run Over by a 1966 Lincoln Continental*, he explains how very much he likes the piece, fondling it ten thousand times before putting it in its box. And he also explains how he made the piece by inking the tires of his father-in-law's car and actually driving right over the piece. The combination of psychological vulnerability coupled with an entirely pragmatic approach is completely characteristic of Westermann.

Turning now to the letter-drawings, we can find them not only an important part of his work but an illuminating source for understanding his sculpture. His genius for drawing manifested itself at an early age. His sister remembers him at the age of eight submitting drawings to the Disney studios. Disney was ready to hire him until they discovered his age. When he was in the Marines during World War II he began the habit of sending drawings and illustrated letters to his family. This practice continued when he moved to Chicago after the war. It is surprising to see how, despite considerable training in commercial and fine art, his very personal drawing style remained intact. Many of the elements of his mature drawing style are already found in his letter-drawings of the fifties, such as an emphasis on contours, words combined with images, a highly compressed narrative structure, a mixture of scales and of perspectives, verbal and visual puns and the use of intense, flatly applied color. Many of these same elements would find a less ephemeral place within the context of his sculpture.

The years 1964-1966 are the most important years for Westermann's letter-drawings. He had married Joanna Beall and in 1961 moved to Brookfield Center, Connecticut where her parents lived. In 1964 Westermann and his wife traveled across the country, settling briefly in San Francisco before moving back to Brookfield Center in 1965. His need to stay in contact with his dealer and his friends, the increased stimulation brought about by travel and new places, both coupled with his desire for creative release may account for the extraordinary flowering of the letter-drawing during this period. Letters such as *Great Cultural Explosion*, *A Country Gone Nuts*, *Suicide Rehearsal* from the section titled **A Country Gone Nuts,** all the letters sent during the trip across the country in **A Tribute to America** and the majority of letters detailing works in progress in the **Sculpture** chapter all date from this period.

In 1968 Westermann went to Tamarind in Los Angeles to produce a suite of lithographs based on his travels called *See America First*. It is about this time that he began to create some watercolors and drawings independent of the letters. He had acquired a sizable reputation for his letter-drawings among his friends and he tried never to disappoint a correspondent, although the burden of keeping up was sometimes difficult. The style of the letters in the early seventies evolves in two areas. He develops an ongoing series of self-caricatures depicting himself in a variety of guises sometimes illustrating a particular event and very often he would repeat the illustration and send it off to a number of different people. The other style of letter-drawing was cross-linked with the watercolors he was working on and usually consisted of abbreviated versions of them with a commentary. Both types of letter-drawing were well-suited to meet the ever-increasing demands made upon him as a correspondent. While they may lack some of the intensity of the letters of the sixties, the drawing style is more accomplished and brings the imaginative power of the last decade of his life into sharp focus.

The letters prove very helpful in explaining what has previously been thought enigmatic in Westermann's work, even though meaning remains in part elusive as indeed Westermann intended. He was never one to disabuse someone of a false interpretation, assuming that if one did not get the idea, no amount of explanations would make a difference. In fact one suspects that Westermann enjoyed covering his tracks and was almost willfully obscure about the sources and meanings in his sculpture.

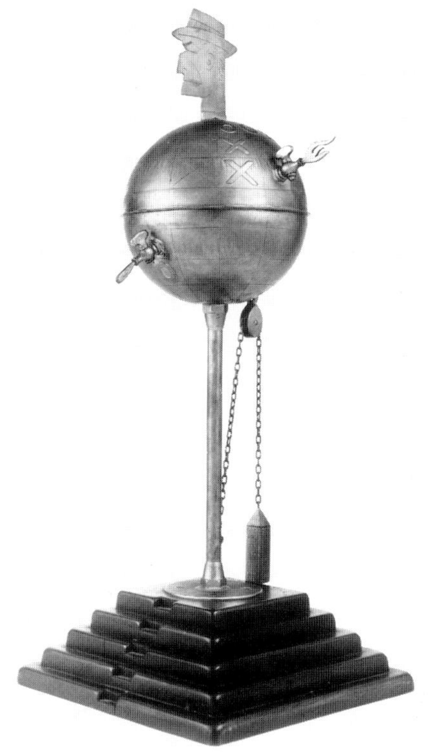

The Unaccountable, collection Betty Asher

An early sculpture, *The Unaccountable* (1959), is a good example of how information from the letters and the chronology in this book can enable us to gain at least partial access to Westermann's work. At first glance the sculpture appears to be a kind of humorous personage. A Dick Tracy head in silhouette sits atop a body made from a toilet tank float on which are incised mercator projection lines which transform it into a globe. A tic-tac-toe game is in progress in the squares formed by the intersection of the lines. Three identical faucets are attached to the body/globe and serve as arms and a penis. One of the faucet arms is closed. Flames emerge from the other arm and from the penis faucet a drop-shaped discharge is frozen in midair. The body/globe is attached to a stepped base by a long thin rod. To the rear of the body, acting as a kind of counterweight to the buoyancy of the torso, is a small office building attached by a chain and pulley. On the base of the building are written the words "Go man go." On the underside of the globe Westermann has soldered a penny and near the flaming spouting faucet is an arrow marked Reno.

If one knows nothing of Westermann's life and understands nothing of the sources, still the piece remains satisfying in its combination of apparently mysterious references. One is amazed by an entirely assured placement of seemingly incongruous parts. However, if one does have access to Westermann's letters and life, it is clear at once that these are in no way random or arbitrary choices. These references do not resolve all the possible meanings inherent in the sculpture into a tidy narrative, but they do serve to animate our understanding of it. Westermann had met and married a singer and dancer named June La Ford whose stage name was Penny Parker during his tour with the USO during 1947. They were separated in 1950 two years after the birth of Westermann's only child Gregory. As a number of letters to his sister Martha as well as titles of early pieces indicate — *I Wonder If I Really Love Her, He Whore, Mysteriously Abandoned New Home* — this was a traumatic experience for Westermann. Then in 1958 he met the love of his life, Joanna Beall, and the letters are full of wonder at his good fortune. She went to Reno in the summer of 1958 to obtain a divorce that cleared the way for their marriage in March of 1959. *The Unaccountable* reverberates with the theme of connection and separation. One cannot simply view this piece as a zany surrealist pop figure. Rather it is a self-portrait commemorating the artist's feelings of hope touched with skepticism at a critical juncture in his life. And by incorporating these literal autobiographical references, private meanings are transformed into public symbols at the intersection of the self and the world.

One of the most curious aspects of the letter-drawings are the elaborate guises that Westermann would assume to project or transform his image. Each phase of his life is represented by a particular self-caricature. We see him as a returning soldier, an acrobat and a young sculptor in Chicago in the form of two idealistic super-heroes, *Mr. Swami* and *Champion of Justice.* He often grafted his features onto the images of characters borrowed from popular culture such as Mickey Mouse, Dick Tracy, Popeye, Santa Claus and Humpty Dumpty. There are also picaresque types such as the *Human Fly*, the *Old Sea Hag*, and the *Blind Captain.* The most common character to emerge in the drawings of the seventies is an aging Romeo in a formal dinner jacket with tails, pomaded hair and patent leather shoes. This can be considered his official portrait, most often shown with gloved hand extended in greeting — a kind of master of ceremonies for the compact narratives of his letters. Westermann's self-projection extended to the animal world as well and the animals with which he chose to identify help explain the nature of his transformations. Included in the bestiary are a rattlesnake, turtle, bat, man-eating shark, vulture, crow, raccoon, pig, a variety of feral-looking dogs and cats and even a cigar-smoking gypsy moth. Sometimes these Westermanns in animal form appear with Westermann in human form engaged in a struggle, as in *Sharks Eating Artists* or *Cliff with Gypsy Moths.* What all these animals share is their status as despised or outcast creatures, beasts needing to be controlled in some way or at least relegated to the margins of the civilized world so that society can function undisturbed.

This tendency toward identification with marginal types is also a feature of some of the most disturbing letters published here. His empathy with subjects who cannot accept or be accepted by society, often ex-seamen or soldiers come to a bad end, is evident in such drawings as *Suicide Rehearsal* where the hanged man has Westermann's tattoo or *Poor Spec* where Westermann displays an odd sympathy with the brutal murderer of eight student nurses in Chicago. In *He's Forgotten about Us* Westermann commemorates the suicide of an anonymous prisoner who escapes confinement and divine indifference by leaping to his death. This is strong stuff indeed, not to be confused with cartoons.

One letter-drawing makes explicit his attitude toward these drawn guises. Across the bottom of a letter showing Westermann as a witch he writes "every time I make a drawing it is a self-portrait." It can be said that all of an artist's production is, no matter how abstract, a self-portrait. However, in Westermann's work the skin that separates his inner and outer selves is unusually thin and permeable. Inner monsters of the subconscious unexpectedly find their way out just as outcasts are able to penetrate in. What makes Westermann unusual as an artist is his ability to so graphically visualize the relationship of the self to the other. The dream-like quality of his imagery and his fertile mixture of word and image suggest the movement of the subconscious outward as it seeks its features in forms that resist limitations imposed by ordinary social and cultural boundaries and so resist easy interpretation. Westermann's art is a celebration of the self's ability to prevail even as it incorporates the outsider into itsélf. Westermann retained his faith in the individual and an optimistic belief in the power and the necessity of art even as he grew increasingly disenchanted with the changes he saw taking place in society as a whole and the art world in particular. The idealism he felt and fought for in World War II was gradually replaced by the conviction that the country had indeed "gone nuts" and was destined to destroy itself through violence and an obsession with materialism. He railed against these things right up to the end of his life leaving us this remarkable legacy to enrich our understanding of his unique contribution to American art.

— Bill Barrette

Early Letters

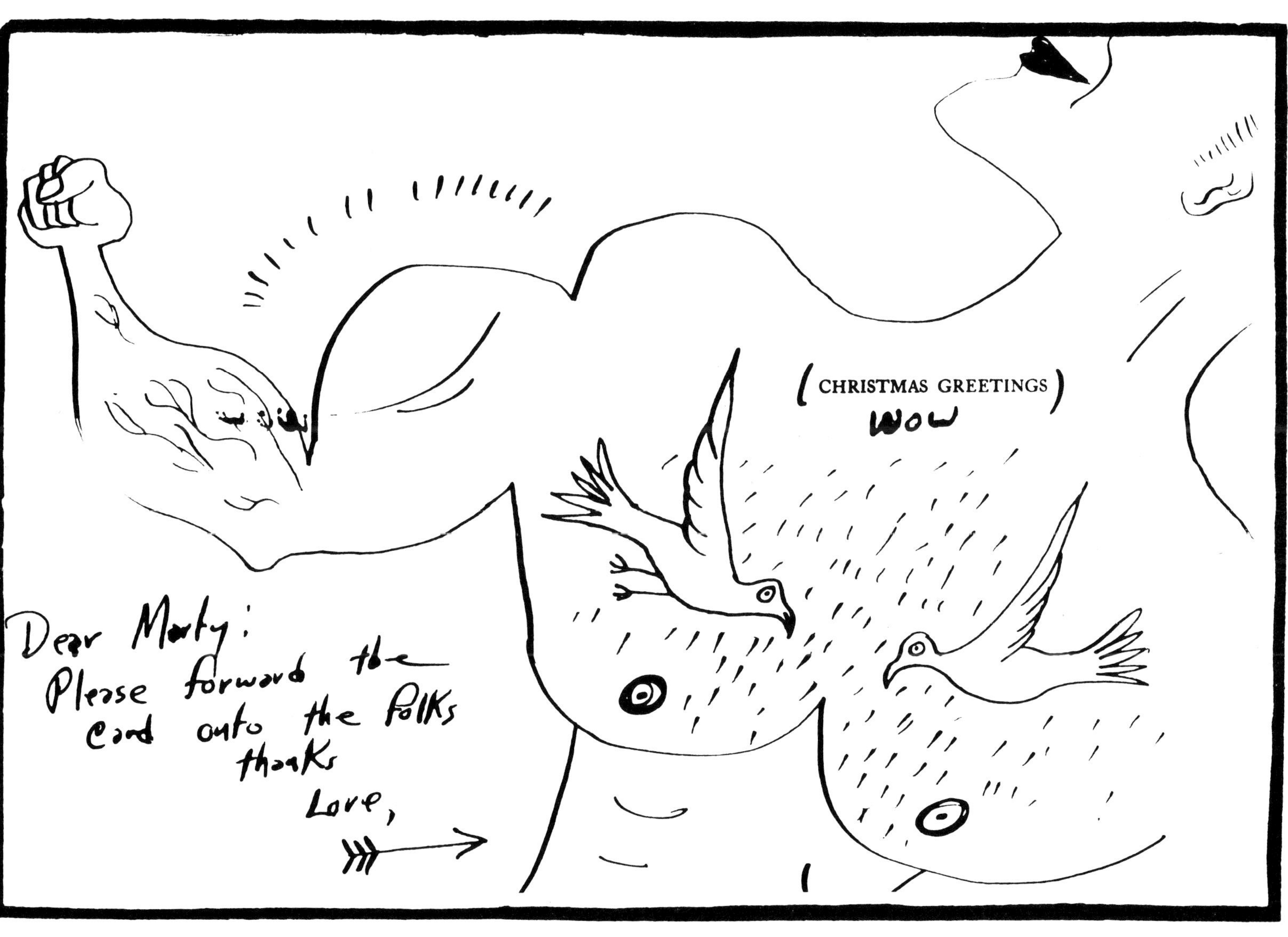

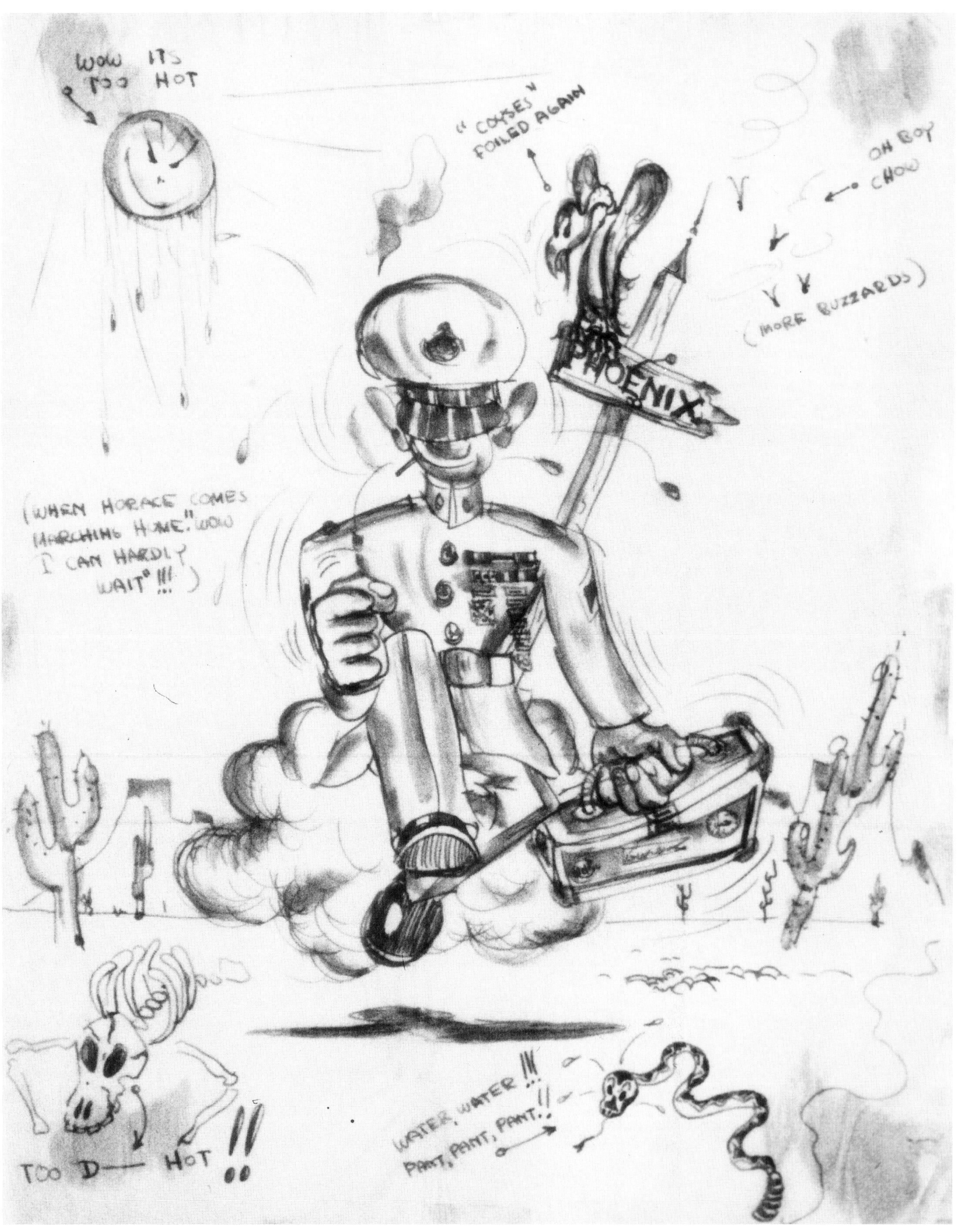
WOW ITS TOO HOT
"CURSES" FOILED AGAIN
OH BOY CHOW
(MORE BUZZARDS)
PHOENIX
(WHEN HORACE COMES MARCHING HOME" WOW I CAN HARDLY WAIT" !!!)
TOO D— HOT !!
WATER, WATER !!! PANT, PANT, PANT !!

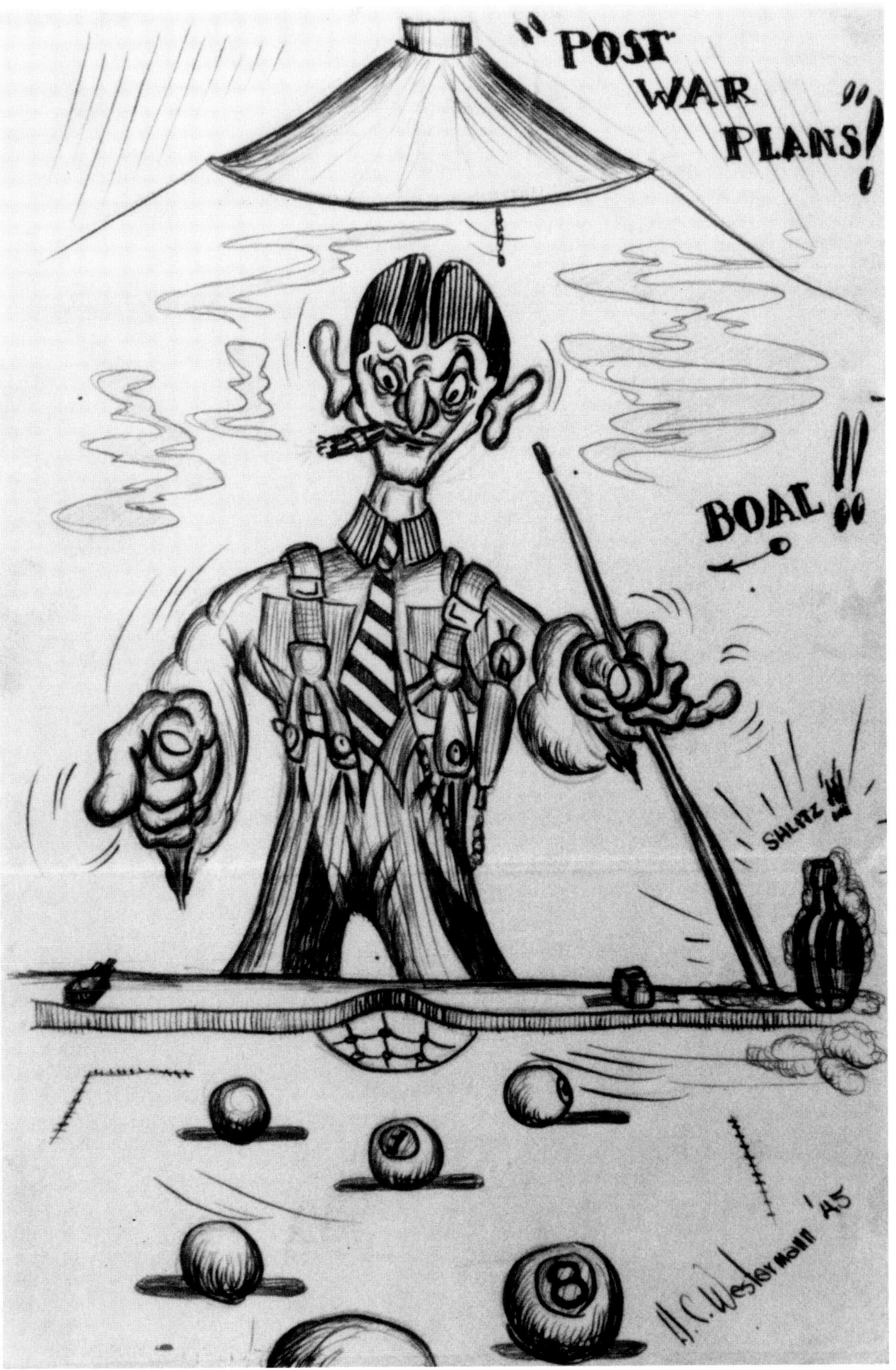
"POST WAR PLANS"!
BOAL!!
SHLITZ
A. C. Westermann '45

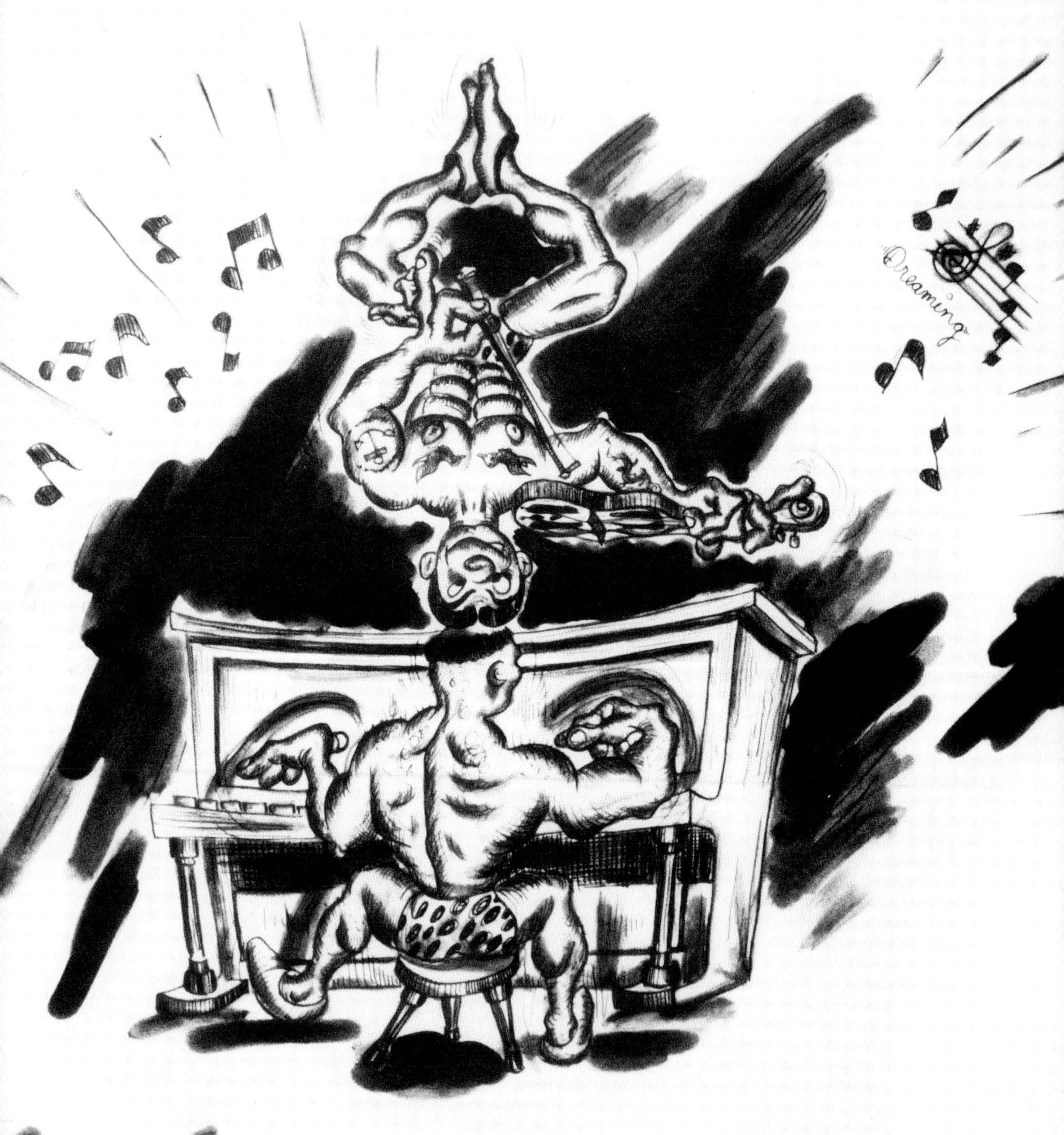
Dreaming
Wayne Westermann
HANDBALANCERS
H.W. 1946

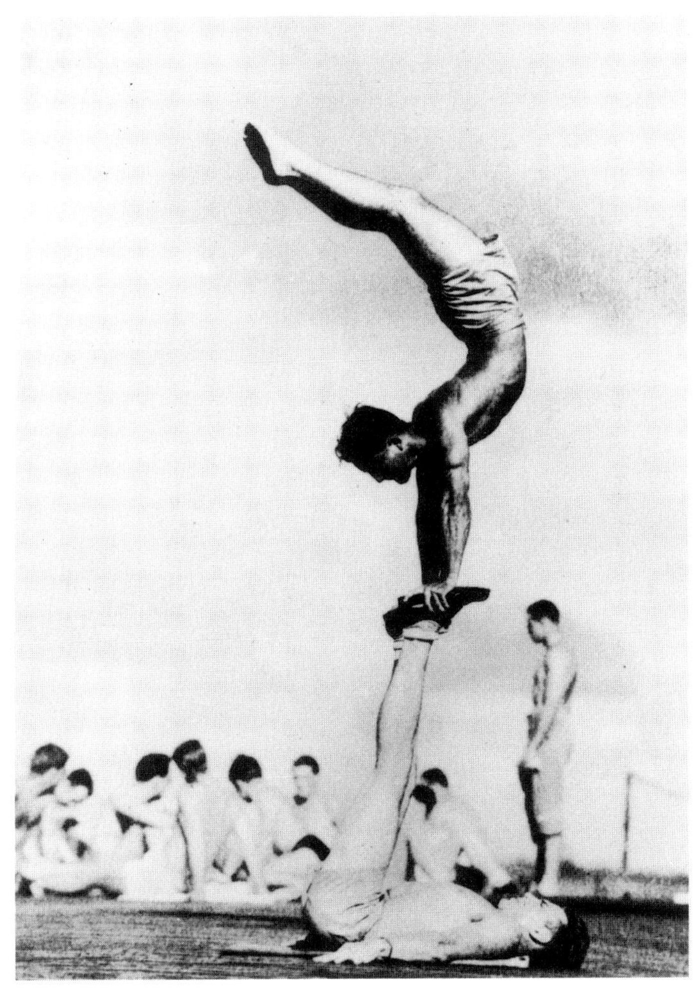

Westermann hand balancing on the USS Enterprise, 1944

from a letter to Barbara Haskell January 11, 1978

When I was an acrobat in showbusiness technically we had a "double handbalancing act." My partner's position or work in the act was that he was the "understander" and I was the "topman." These are the correct terms for describing our act and as you know we were on a U.S.O. tour of the Orient for 1 year '46-'47.

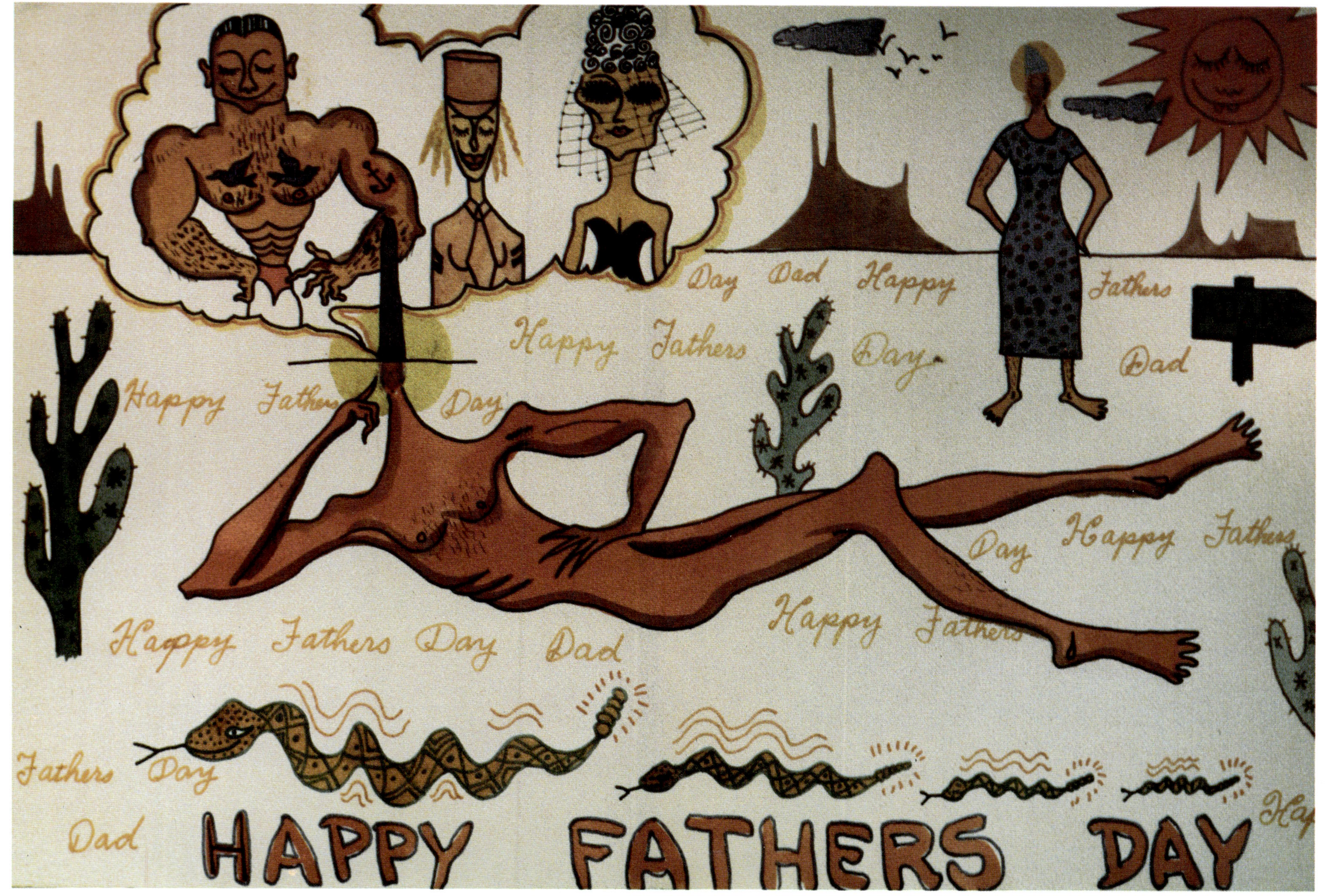
HAPPY FATHERS DAY

October 14, 1976

Dear Martha + Mike:

It was good to get your letter + sorry to hear you have to go back to night school — that must make it rough, because you are so involved in so many things. I don't know how you do it all? That amazes us. I was sure sorry to hear Penny + Joe broke up. I really like both of them. Give her my regards.

Dad was a good soldier + always covered his tracks, so to speak, + he was quiet. On the other hand, there are the big loud mouths. Martha, Dad was a very successful person — (+ real success has very little, if nothing, to do with money). He was a very highly respected person in his profession + was probably the best. During the Depression when hundreds of accountants were out of work he managed to keep his job + mainly because he was an asset to Horwath + Horwath + he was honest + had great integrity. In terms of money he was worth a lot more to that company than he ever got. He put his family above himself + allowed himself to be exploited + of course by doing that he had to let his "Great Expectations" go down the drain — + he had Great Expectations! So his energy went into doing the best possible job at his work + he tried + willed his work to be his expression. Under those circumstances he had "class," which most people don't understand or are even aware of — + he had "guts" of a nature that could easily be miscomprehended. Well he was an unsung hero.

Another unsung hero was our gramma Bloom. I think she was another completely underestimated person. She had a lot of character. She was a gentle + kind person. Do you know during the Depression she carried quite a few of those tenants in her court, when they couldn't pay the rent. I remember many Saturdays I used to go over there + spend the day. Well I loved her company + I'd usually be working at a model airplane at her dining room table all day + she respected that I was sensitive + never, never, interrupted me, you know to stop + ask me to do little shit details for her. Nor would she start chatting when I was busy. She was always very quiet + we both enjoyed each other's company. She was really a fine fine woman + those Saturdays meant a lot to me. She was nice to everybody.

Martha, the last time we were in L.A. I went back to Norwich Dr. + you know there's just nothing there anymore — I mean where our home used to be. Well that was a traumatic experience. It was like we had never had a home or a family or been even been born — none of us. I think its awful the things they do + once around is enough for me.

Love,
Cliff

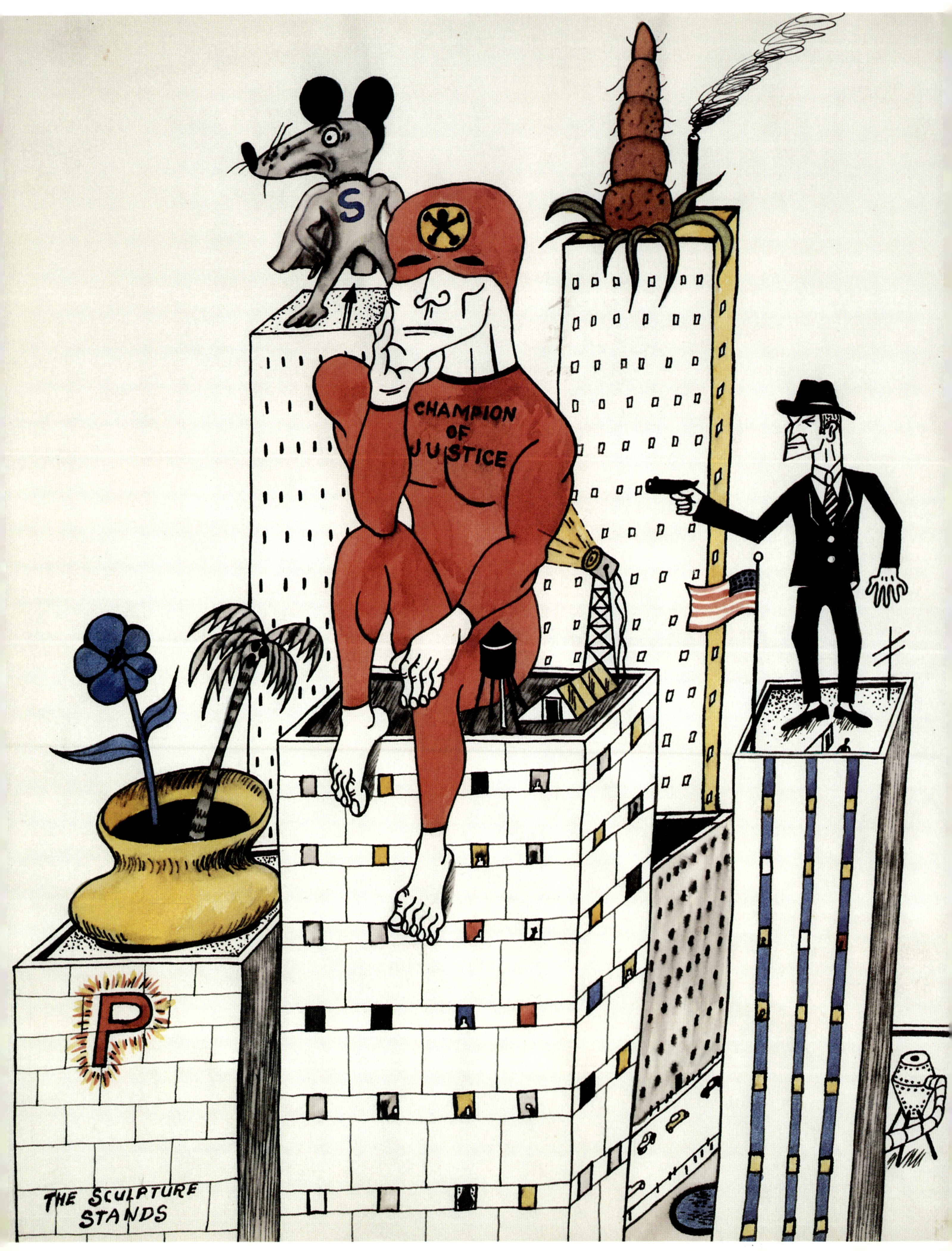
S
CHAMPION OF JUSTICE
P
THE SCULPTURE STANDS

September 20, 1958

Dear Martha + Mike:

I've thought of you three a good deal + it's been a long time since I've written. I'm sorry, I know I owe you a letter or two. I have been working exceedingly hard over quite an extended period of time now + I'm a little beat. It's about time for another month in Frisco. I hope I can make it again this year, we'll see. I've an idea you are in your new home now + good luck. How about a little snapshot. How's little Heidi? I'll bet she's quite a little doll now + how are all your wires and strange machines Mike. Don't get em crossed. Since I got back from out there it's been a good + productive period even though it's been difficult financially + otherwise. The pieces get harder + more complex, which actually I welcome, as here is where the real adventure is. In art you are a great adventurer in a sense that you can enter frontiers never before explored by anyone + it's quite exciting + mysterious. The responsibility that art requires is unimaginable, even to most artists oddly enough. But of course the sheer satisfaction could not be bought for any price. I'm really very grateful to be a practitioner of this great, wonderful, mysterious, intangible. Actually there are perhaps a half dozen people that I talk art with so forgive me for maybe beating you to death. I think sometimes people write to get things off their chest or to express some things sometimes. Maybe this is an insincere motive. Regardless I do love you very much — the three of you + you were so fine to me when I was there last time. I've thought of it many times + its like the first breath of spring. Thank you ever so much again even though I didn't go out of my way one bit for you. I'm real bad in some respects + I'm quite aware of it + just never seem to change. My personal life is still a mess + grows worse progressively, ha, ha. I guess I'm relegated to always walking this tightrope, but this is the way it has to be. It's the only way I can live + get my work done. Do you know today I have one dollar in the bank + three cents in my pocket + I'm a pretty happy man + not worried a bit. Next week I'll have a few bucks again. Seems I'm always spending my last nickel on a piece of wood or glue or a tool + I don't worry. I have a roof over my head + eat + I only owe ten dollars altogether + generally I have the time I need which is the most important thing. I think this letter is doing me more good than it will you, ha, ha. This one is like talking to a close friend so just bear me a while. I feel if I can keep creating the time as I've done I'll be doing some <u>real</u> fine things someday. It's not the ones behind you that excite you as it is the prospect of the ones you're going to do. However I get maybe too excited doing them generally. But then can a man give <u>too</u> much of himself to his work?? I don't think so. I would most certainly prefer to die than do one, just one, piece that I didn't pour everything conceivable within me, into. And this I mean right from my heart. Art is not to be cheated or bargained with as are business practices and art is pretty brutal when it is not respected or the improper insight is shown. And yet somehow I am certainly not afraid of it, on the contrary, I want more more than anything to come to grips with it — with a clear conscience + with courage + strength. Oh how I love it.

In a sense each piece is a reassurance of my own inner self true inner self that is. So many things to uphold. The idea of art itself is so beautiful it thrills me to write this sentence. Well I've spent my paper talking about myself. I suppose I should apologize, but I really had to write this letter. + I do love you three. Tell everybody in Sacramento hello + kiss La Nore for me.

Love,
Cliff

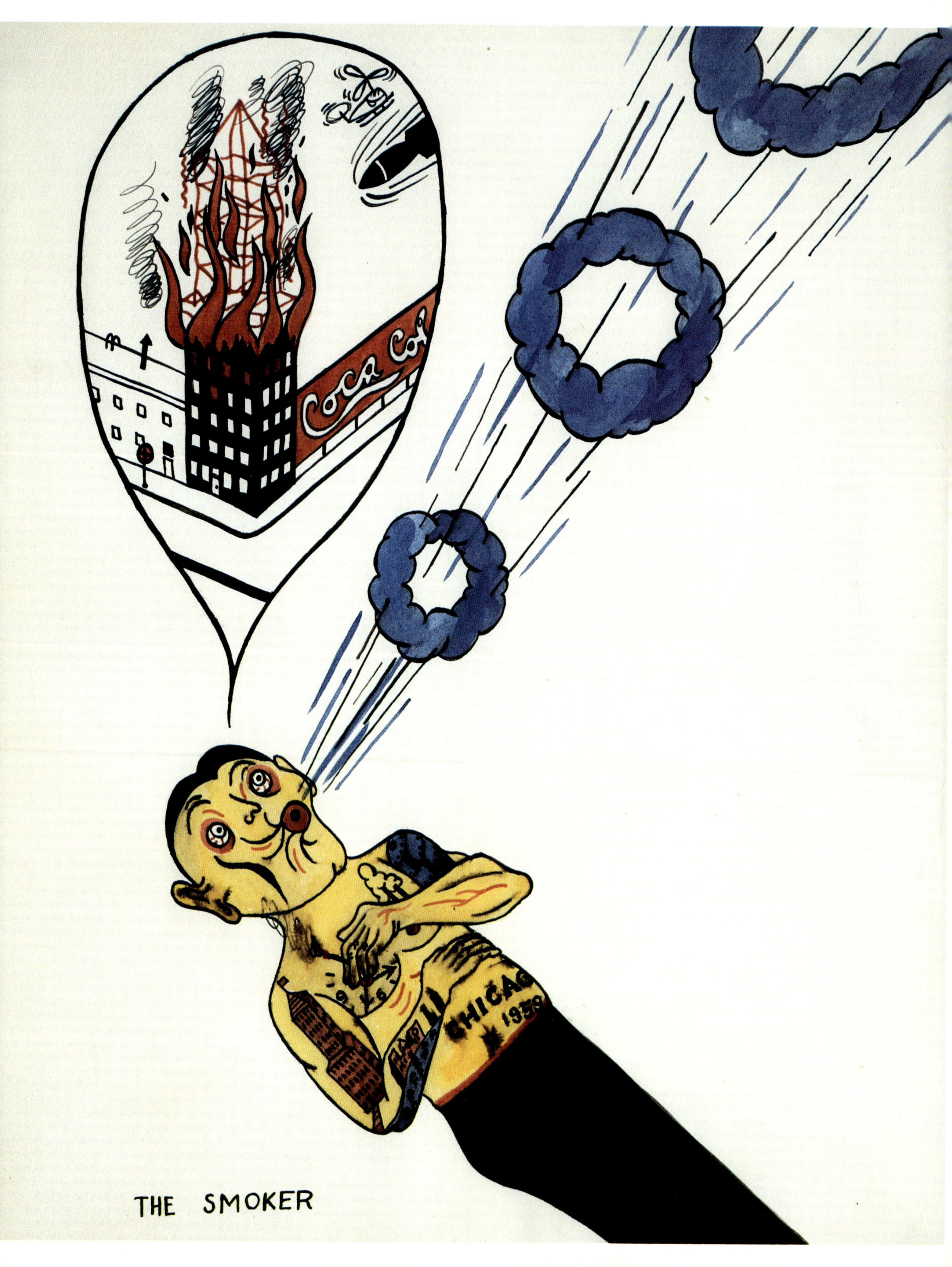
Coca Col
CHICAG
THE SMOKER

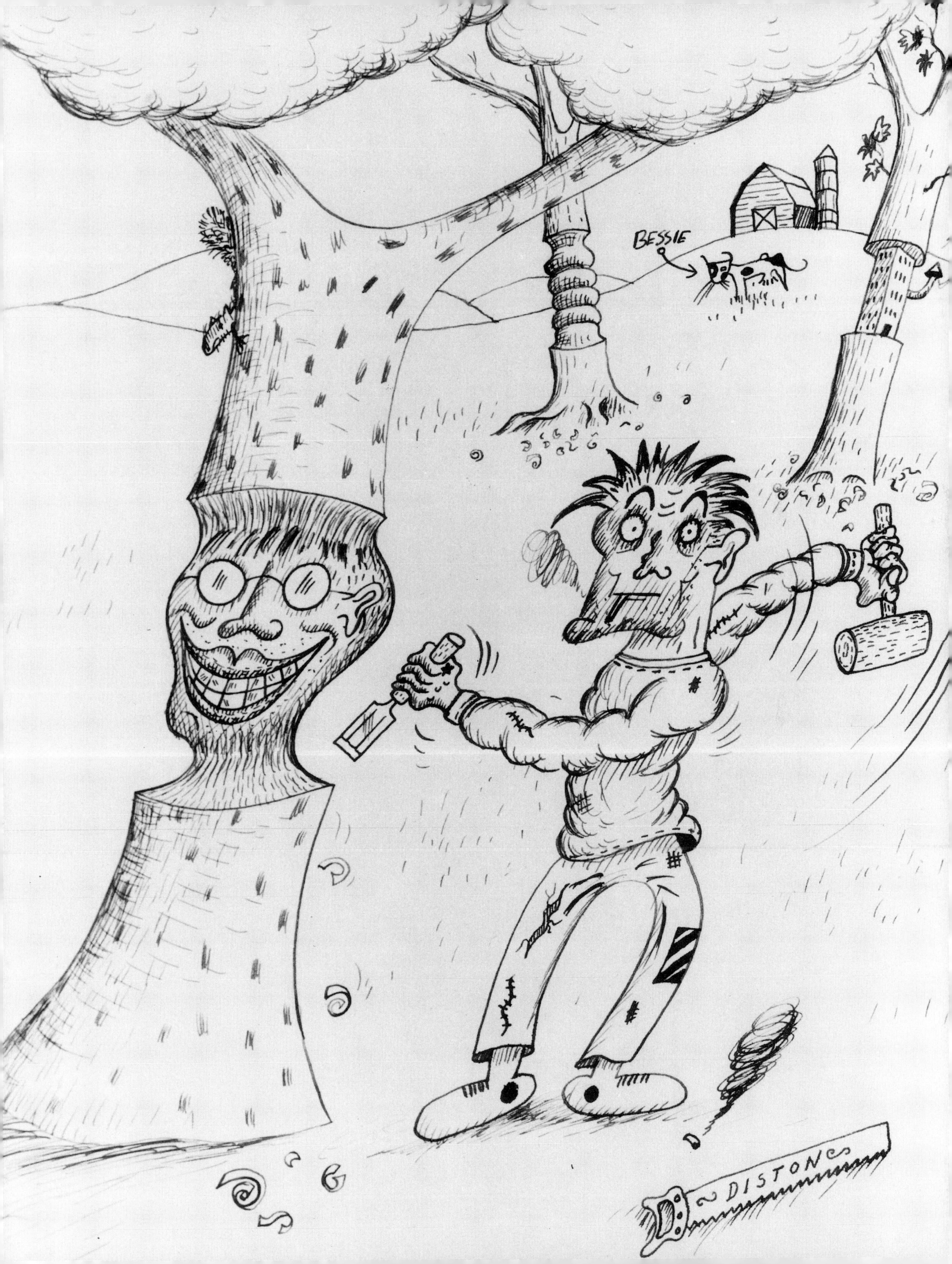
BESSIE
DISTON

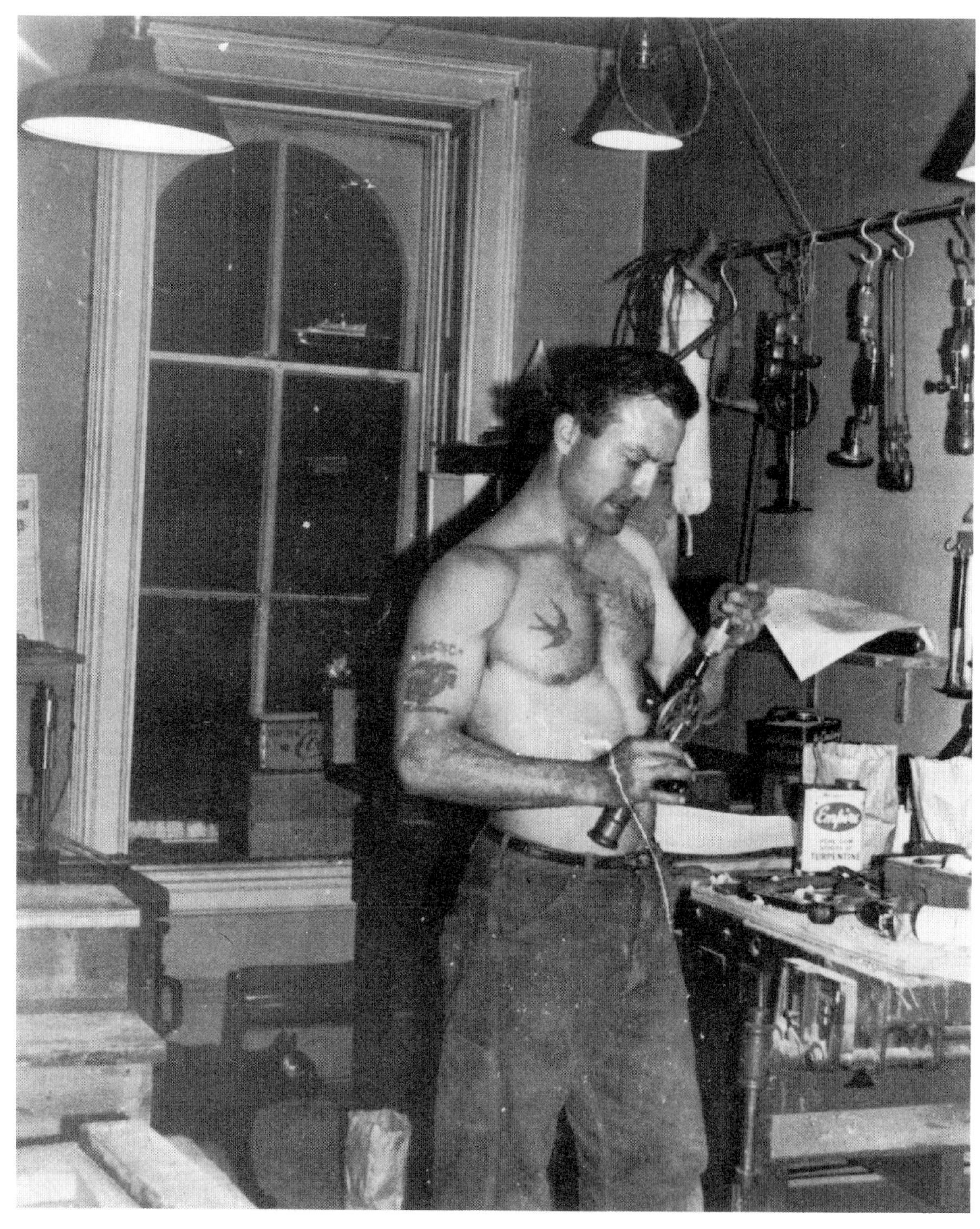

Westermann in his studio at 222 North Avenue, Chicago, 1960

February 24, 1959

Dear Martha and Mike:

Hi—How are you and how's the new house? I hope you're well settled + very happy by now. Soon it will be a year since you moved. Things here happened fast and furious lately and have changed considerably. For one I'm getting married soon and tonight Joanna and I are leaving for Mexico (Yucatan Peninsula) for a month or two. She's a wonderful person and I've been going with her now for over a year. We're very close and she's a fine fine artist. We share the same interests and are very happy together. I've never been happier in my life. Oh yes, too, we understand completely our individual problems as artists. We'll come and visit sometime, soon I hope. I know she'll like you and you her. The show is well underway and Allan is very excited etc. Next year five of the pieces will be in a very important show at the Mus. of Modern Art in N.Y. So I feel very lucky etc. However time and just being fortunate to work is the greatest gift of all. I shy from all those social functions, etc. connected with showings etc. I certainly never realized a year ago all this would happen and up til Christmas I was penniless and things were pretty grim, but I was happy because I was working. Now I really need another rest and so does she as we've both worked very hard up til now. I think of you often and love you and relive S.F. occasionally. It was very pleasant and a much needed rest. Somehow Joanna's been a tremendous influence and loving her has been such a boost, extremely understanding and she doesn't mind poverty and doesn't want for very many things. What a doll, and she's very beautiful too. Give my regards to the Blooms and La Nore and I love you.

Cliff

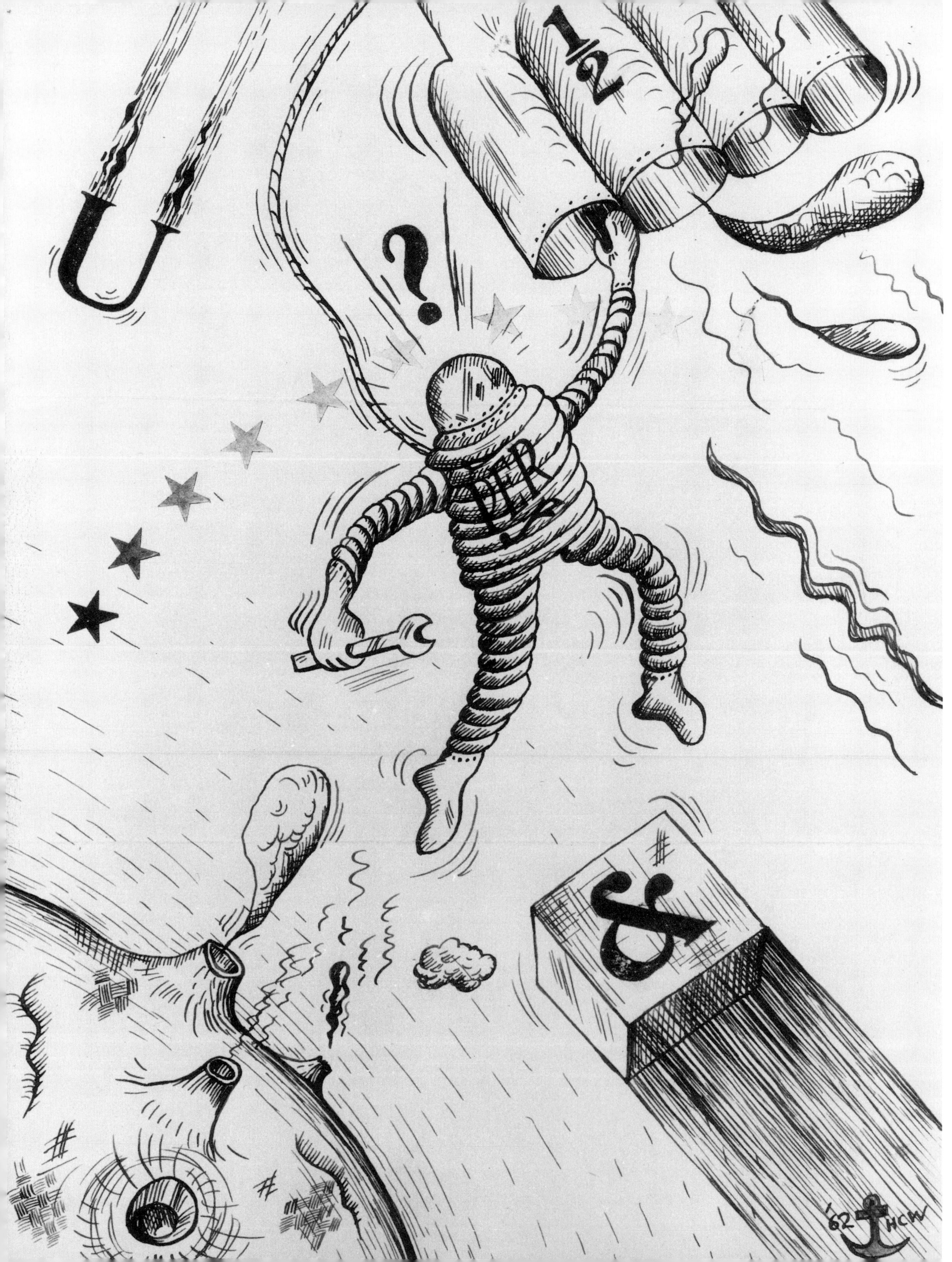
½
PER
'62 HCW

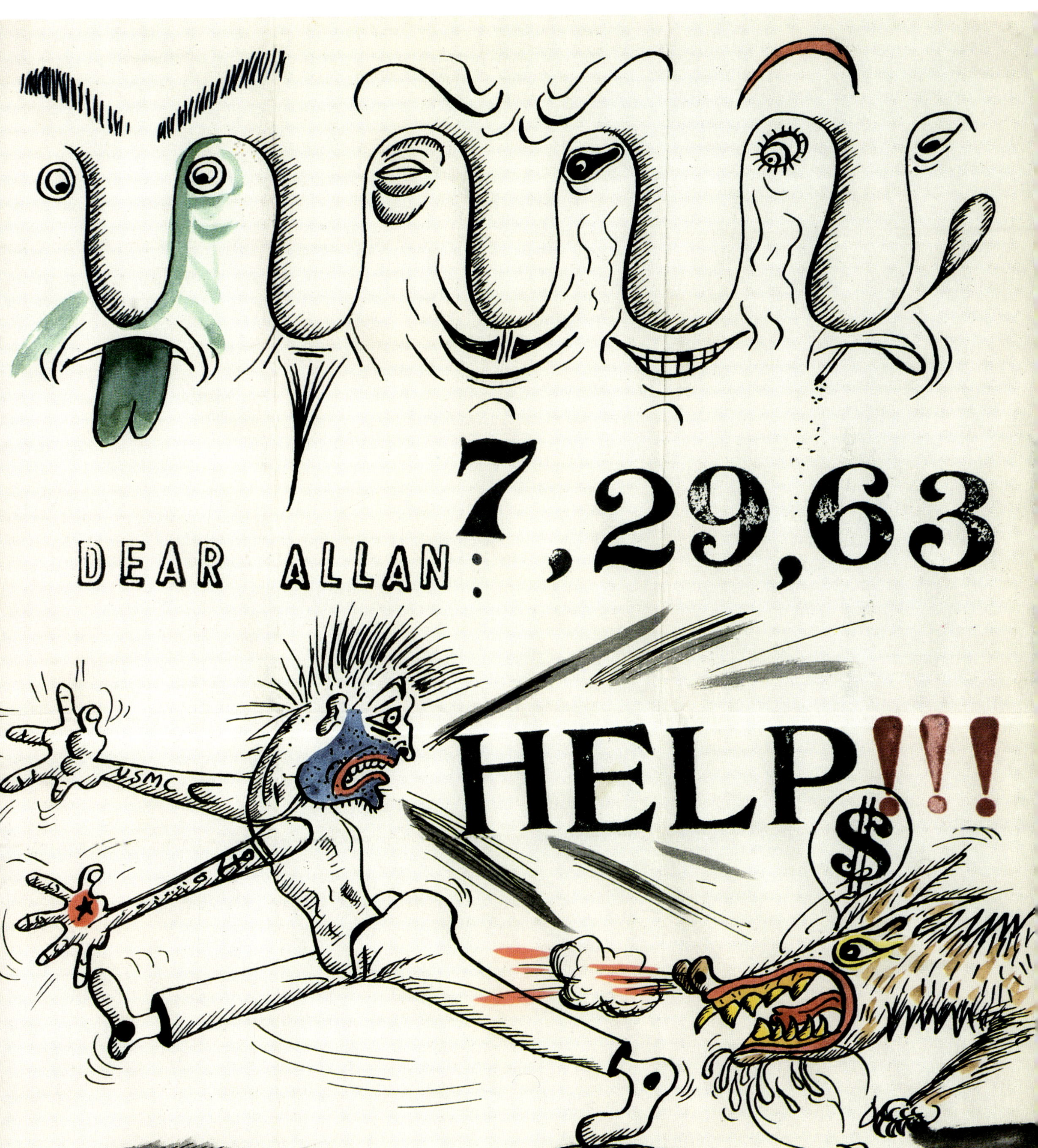
DEAR ALLAN: 7,29,63
HELP!!!
USMC
$

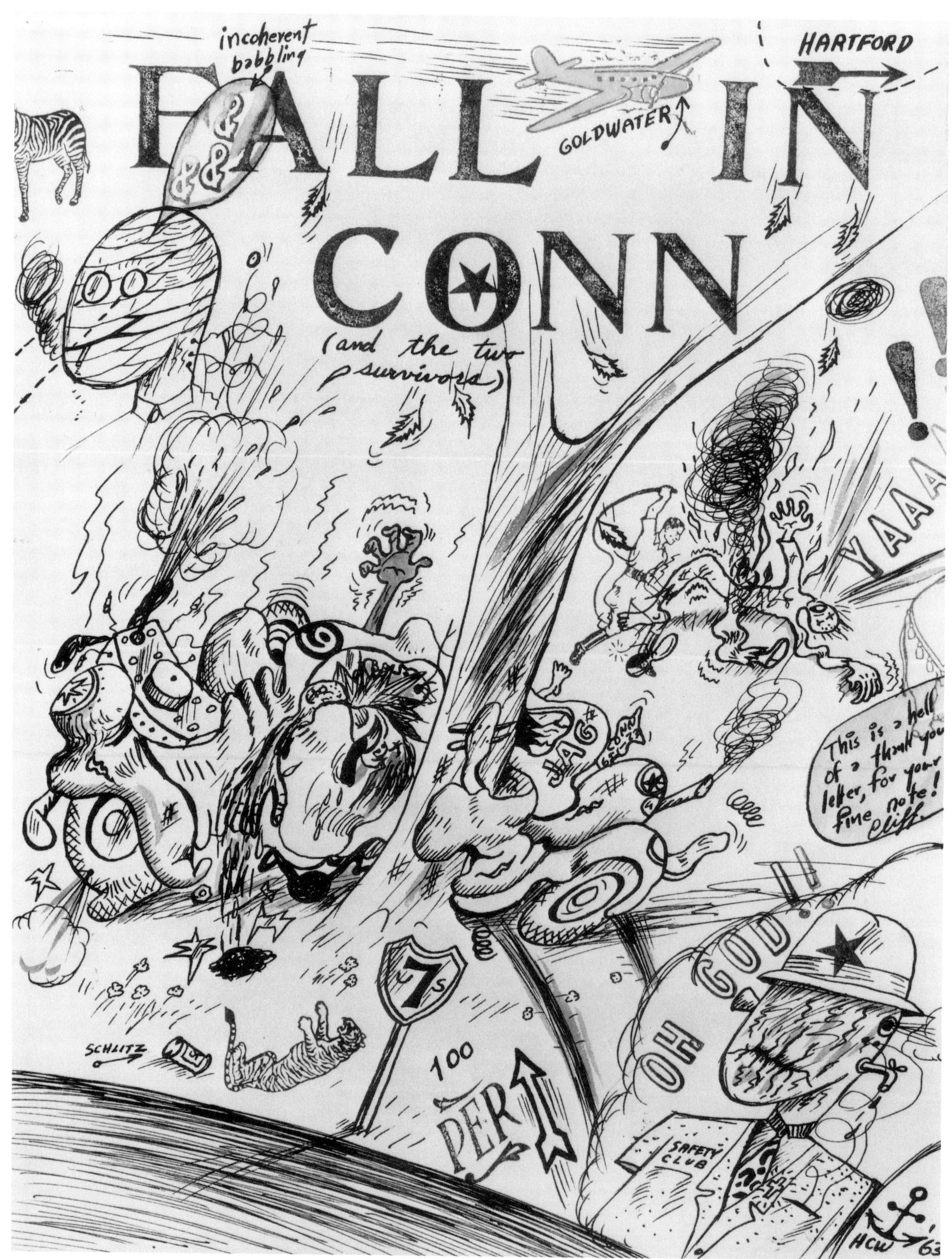
incoherent babbling
HARTFORD
GOLDWATER
FALL IN CONN
(and the two survivors)
YAAAA!!
This is a hell of a thank you letter, for your fine note! Cliff
OH GOD!!
SCHLITZ
7
100
PER
SAFETY CLUB
HCW 63

April 27, 1964

Dear Martha and Mike:

We received your fine letter + are always glad to hear from you. Thanks. Things sound very normal there. I'll bet you will be glad when the house is finished. That sure has been a big job. This (*referring to illustration in the right hand margin*) is a huge willow tree down in the field from our cottage + it is very yellow now + soon the leaves will become green. They are beautiful trees but are not very structural. Last fall a wasp became trapped in my shop + I kept him alive all winter by feeding him sugar water + then a couple of weeks ago when the weather got warmer, he got the call + left. I think this was quite amazing. He actually got to know me + look for his sugar water, + we became great pals. But he had to go. And I could get very near him + he never minded. Joanny sold a fine piece of hers to a very good collector in N.Y. It was a beauty. We are looking for a large covered truck now and intend to move out there sometime this summer probably. We hope. We have just about "run out of gas" here. We still have a little more work however + then packing. You know. How are the artist kids? I love their drawings you know. Joanny has been some wonderful paintings lately. I think she is one of the finest artists in the country. I sure love that girl + we are also great pals, + have so much fun together. And she's a terrific sculptor.

You know the N.Y. art scene is about the phoniest thing there is. Its a joke + its fantastic how many of them "pirate" from other artists. In Chicago in 1954 I had a terrific technical problem with a piece I was working on + I was very broke. I had some beautiful ¾" maple shelves that I had gotten from a carpentry job I had. Well I devised my system of laminating + solved my problem + from this technique I developed + finally went on to laminating ¾" plywood + for very good reasons. Well since then in the N.Y. art magazines I have read articles by artists about how they invented laminating + since 1960, ha ha. But these people, + I have seen their work, have never used it right. They use it decoratively which is horrible. So that's the way it works. I have never stolen from another artist + if I had I would certainly give the artist credit.

And then you have the cheap gossip amongst the artists + critics that is devastating — literally horrible lies. Oh boy this is really vicious. Last year I had (a very bad) critic call me a has been "playboy". For some reason this guy hates me + I've never met him. Joanny + I work constantly + go to a party about once a year. This is a joke. These critics love to attack you personally (which has nothing to do with your work). Its horrible!! My own work + destiny I can control but these horrible politics + "brown nosing" + gossip is beyond me. I hate it. Well this is about the size of it. They all attend too many parties and don't work. Well all my love anyway + I think of you.

Love,
Cliff

Tribute to America

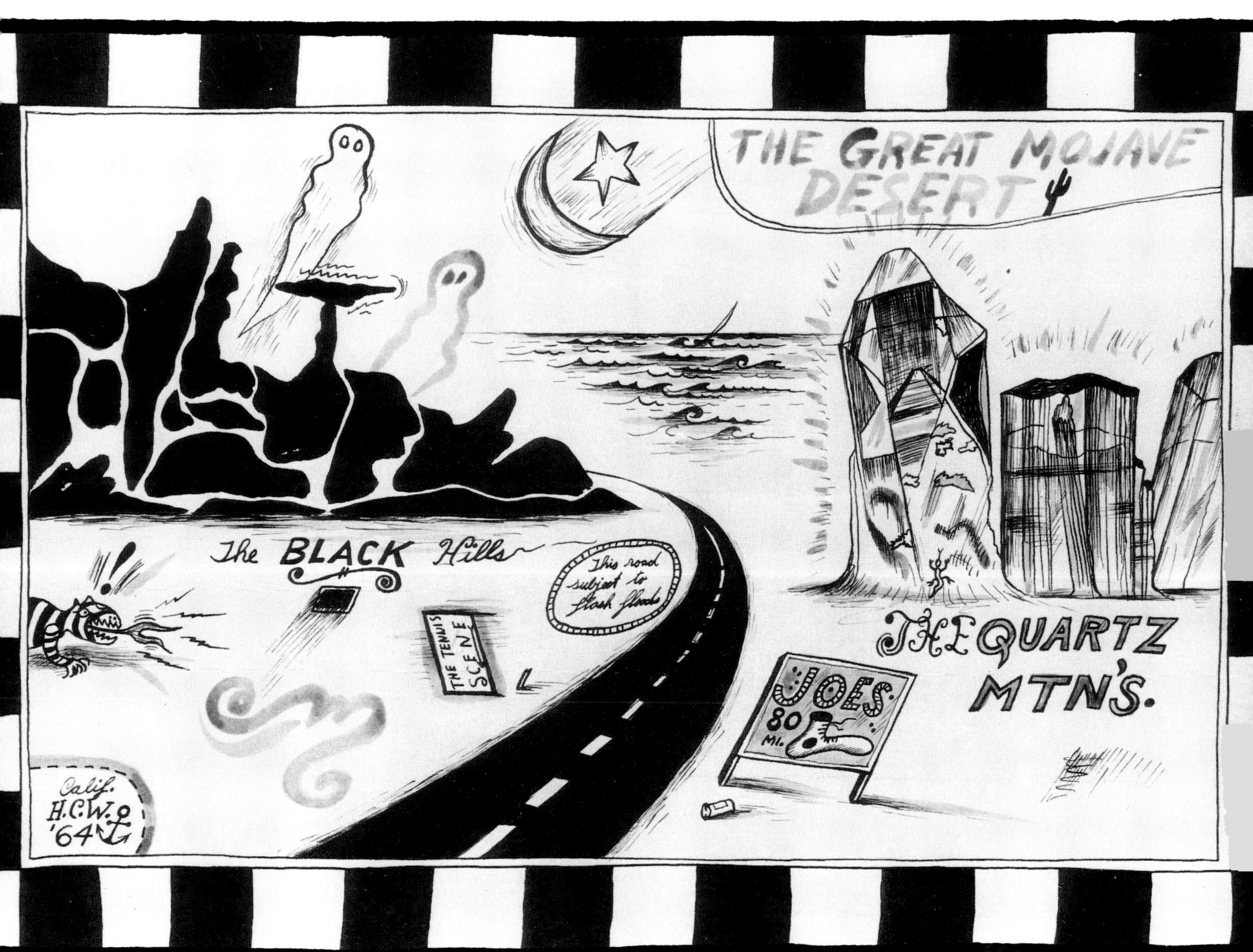

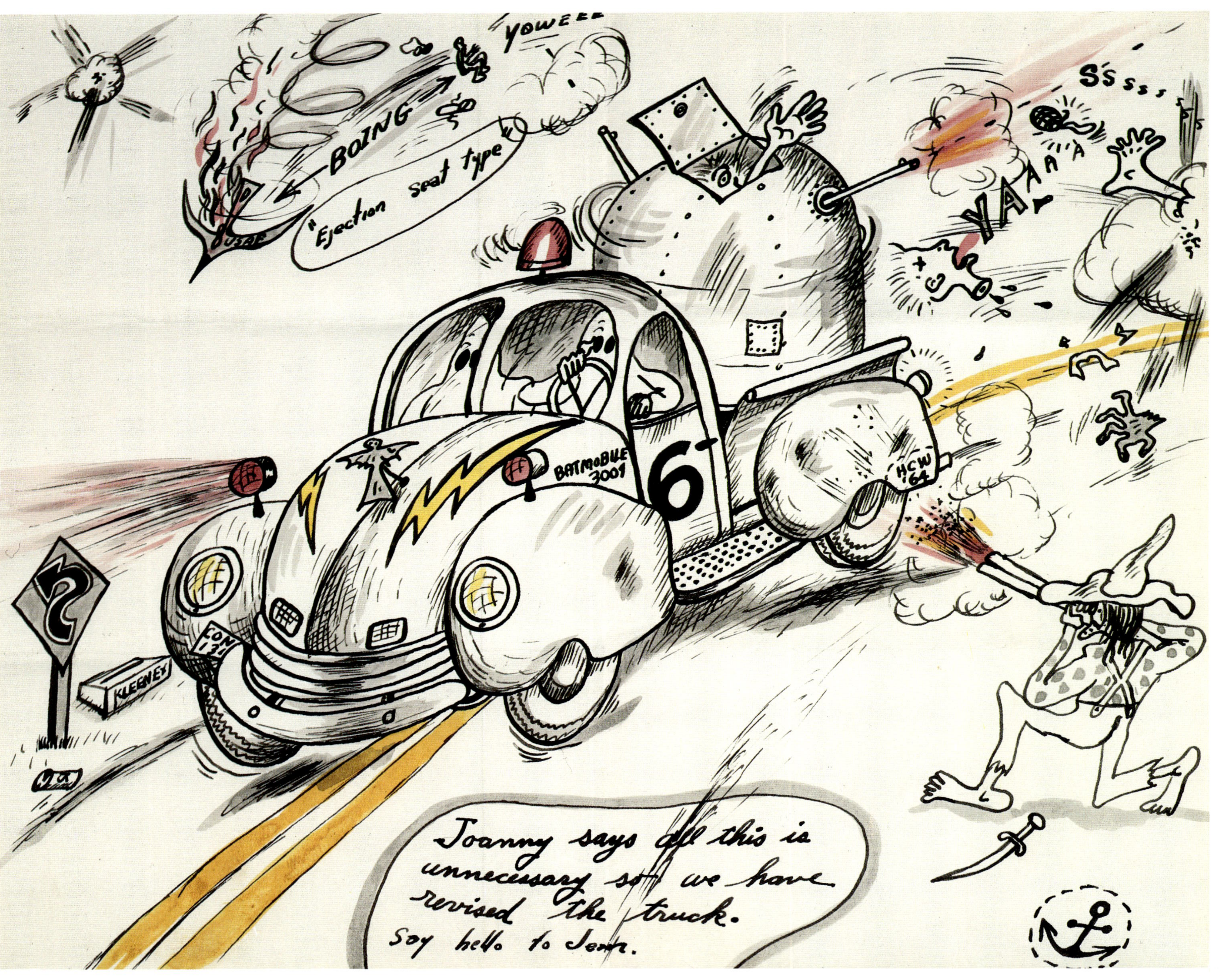
YOWEEE
BOING
"Ejection seat type"
SSssss
YAAAA
BATMOBILE 3001
6
HCW 64
KLEENEX
Joanny says all this is unnecessary so we have revised the truck.
Say hello to Jean.

from a letter to Allan Frumkin June 29, 1964

WELL we bought a 1950 Chevy pick up truck + have been working like hell on it. We've had it a little over a week now + it's coming along. We love it. Here is our plan. We are fixing up the truck so we can live in the back part + are going out to Calif. (about latter July) + just look around good from L.A. up to S.F. + try to get a place. Then if we find a place we'll leave the little truck there, take a bus back here, rent a big truck, load all our stuff on it + drive out there for good. This is going to take a little time, but we think this is the best plan. We are having a lot of fun too. It's good to get away from pieces for now. I know when we get settled + I go back to work, the pieces will be better than ever.

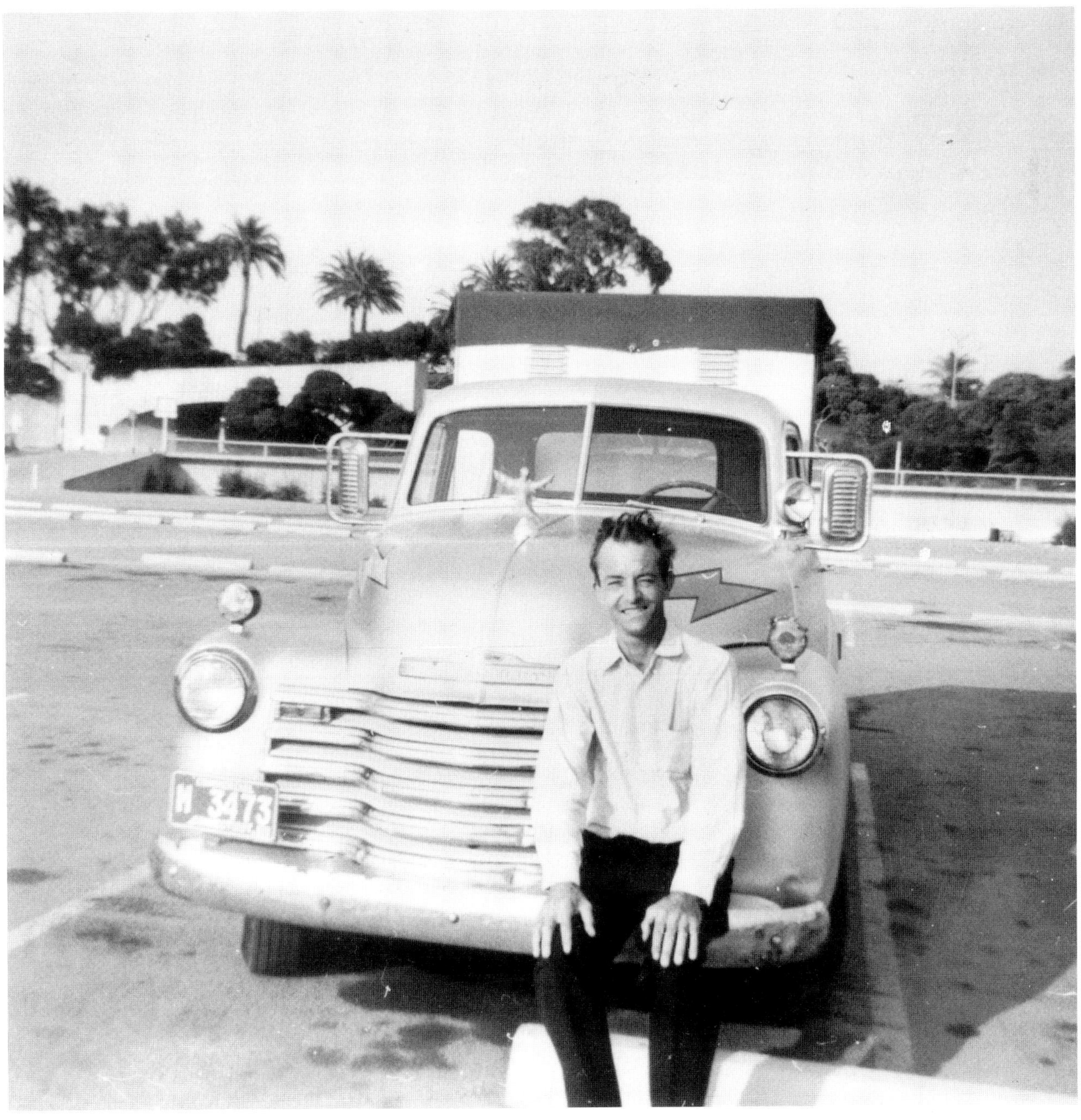

Westermann in front of the Batmobile in Los Angeles, 1964

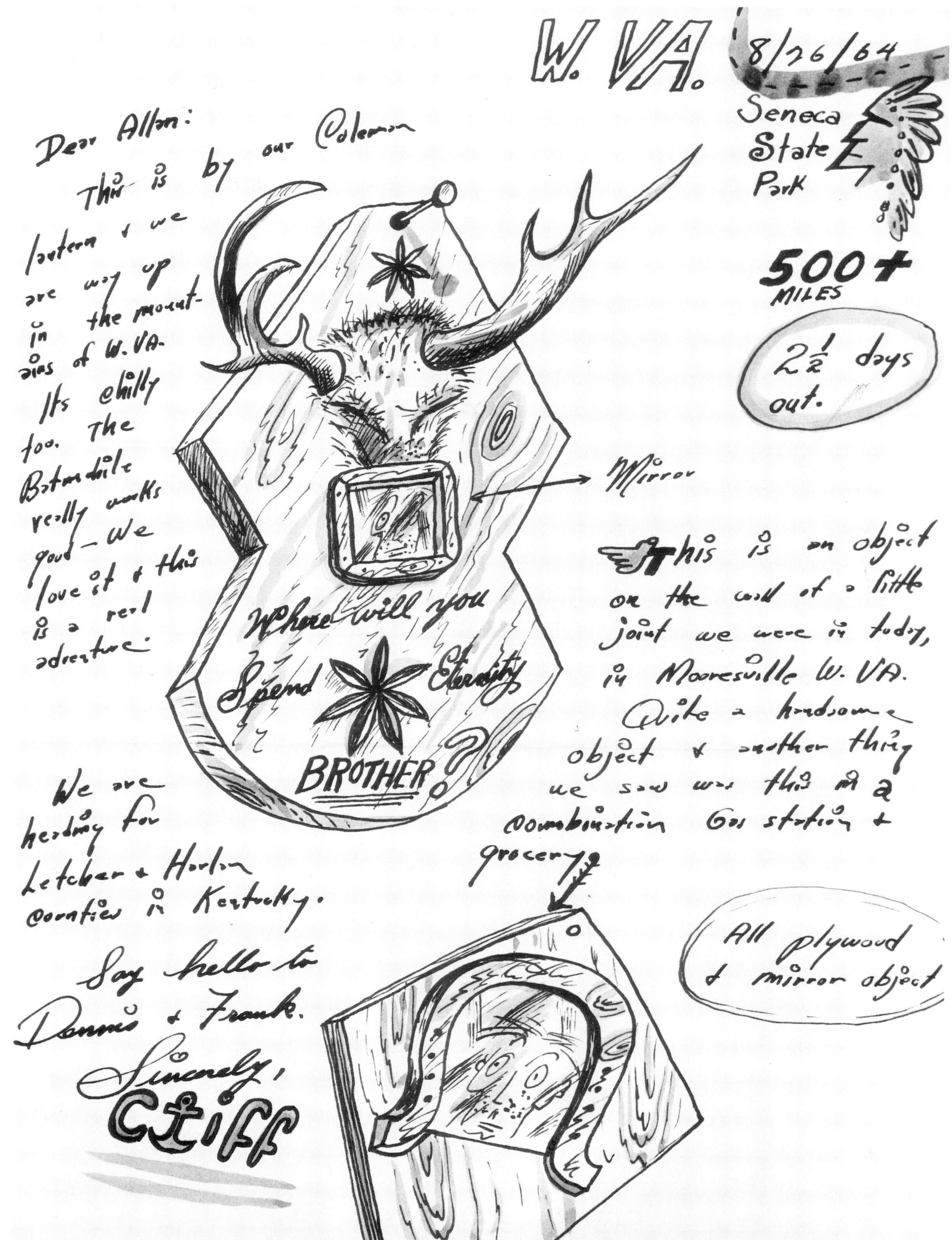

W. VA. 8/26/64

Seneca State Park

500+ MILES

2½ days out.

Dear Allan:

This is by our Coleman lantern & we are way up in the mountains of W. VA. Its chilly too. The Batmobile really works good — We love it & this is a real adventure.

This is an object on the wall of a little joint we were in today, in Mooresville W. VA. Quite a handsome object & another thing we saw was this in a combination Gas station & grocery.

All plywood & mirror object

We are heading for Letcher & Harlan counties in Kentucky.

Say hello to Dennis & Frank.

Sincerely,

Cliff

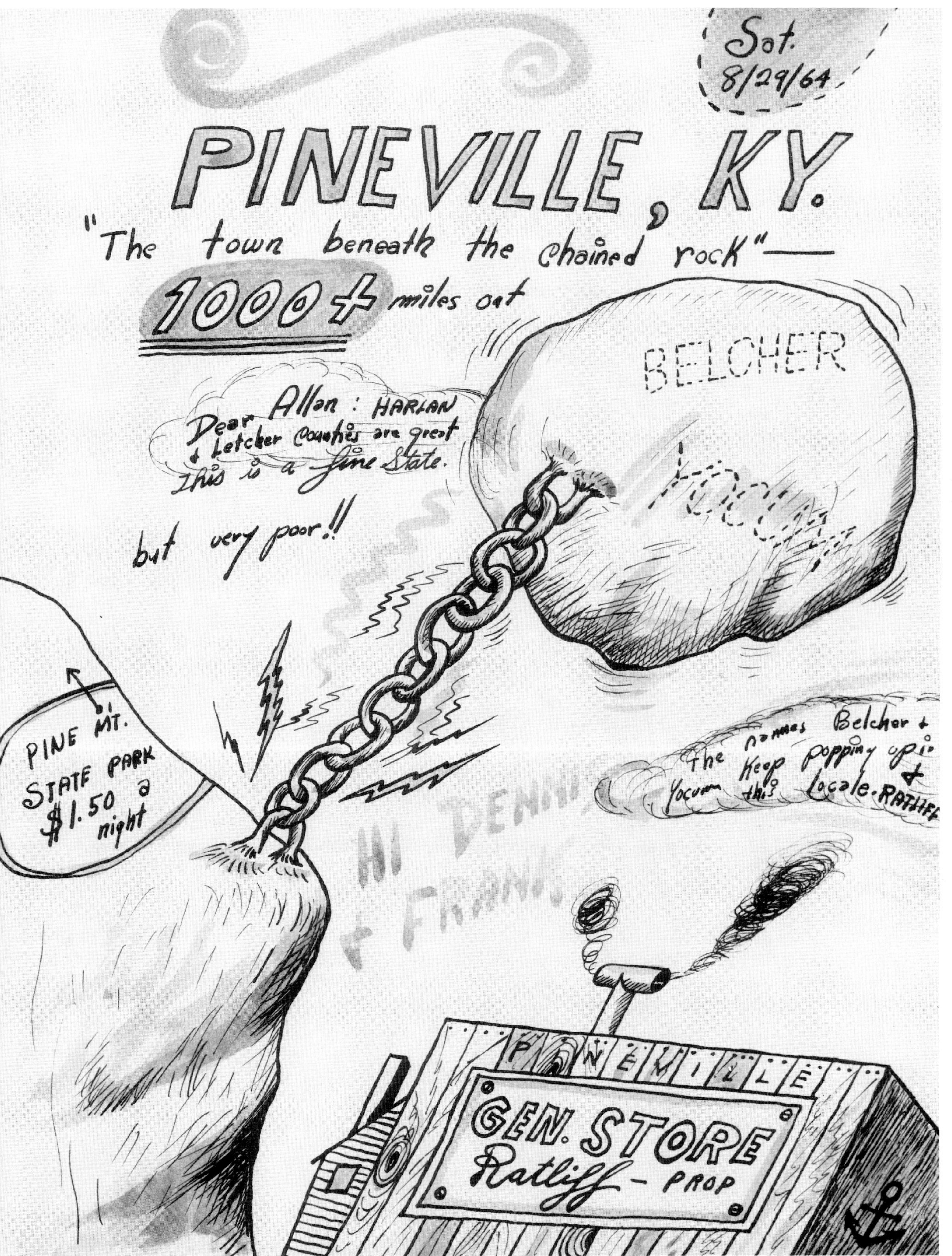
Sat.
8/29/64
PINEVILLE, KY.
"The town beneath the chained rock"—
1000+ miles out
BELCHER
YOCUM
Dear Allan: HARLAN & Letcher Counties are great
This is a fine State.
but very poor!!
PINE MT. STATE PARK
$1.50 a night
The nammes Belcher &
Keep popping up in
Yocum this Locale. RATLIF
&
HI DENNIS
& FRANK
PINEVILLE
GEN. STORE
Ratliff - PROP

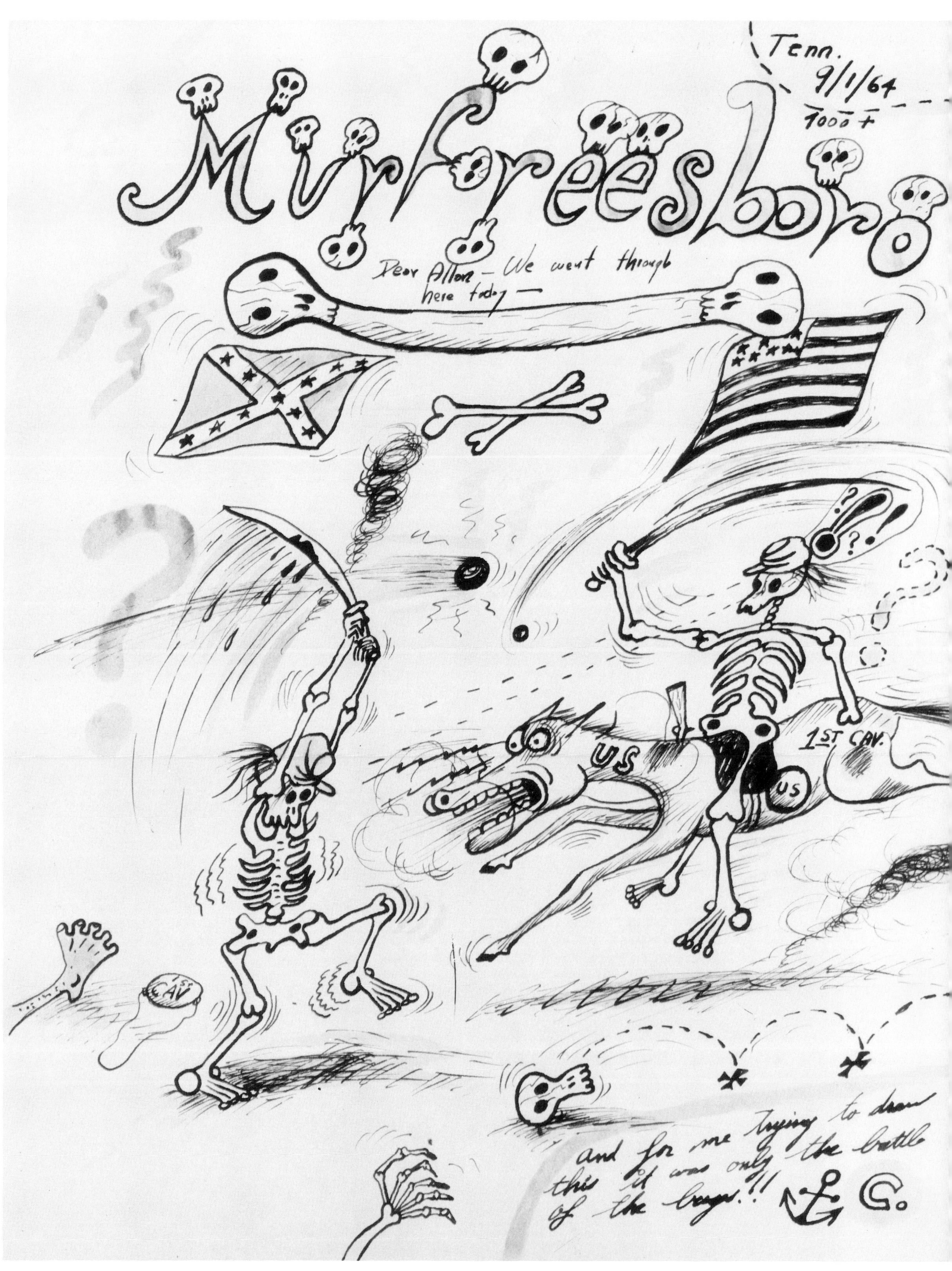
Murfreesboro
Tenn.
9/1/64
1000+
Dear Allen — We went through here today —
US
1ST CAV.
US
1ST CAV
And for me trying to draw the battle
this it was only
of the boys!!
G.

HOTEL ANTLER JACKSON, TENN. 9/1/64

Dear Allan: We had to stop over a day here to have the truck fixed & in the hotel lobby was this pts of 80 year old man had made & given the proprietress. Corrugated cardboard & the same glued on as to frame. ✉ — Collage & painting —

I might add that Cox's raid was here in 1862. Apparently this was a northern GARRISON.

ESSO
HUMBLE
HAPPY MOTORING
36
32
30

This ole man was here dying in the hospital — I don't know his name.

L.C.

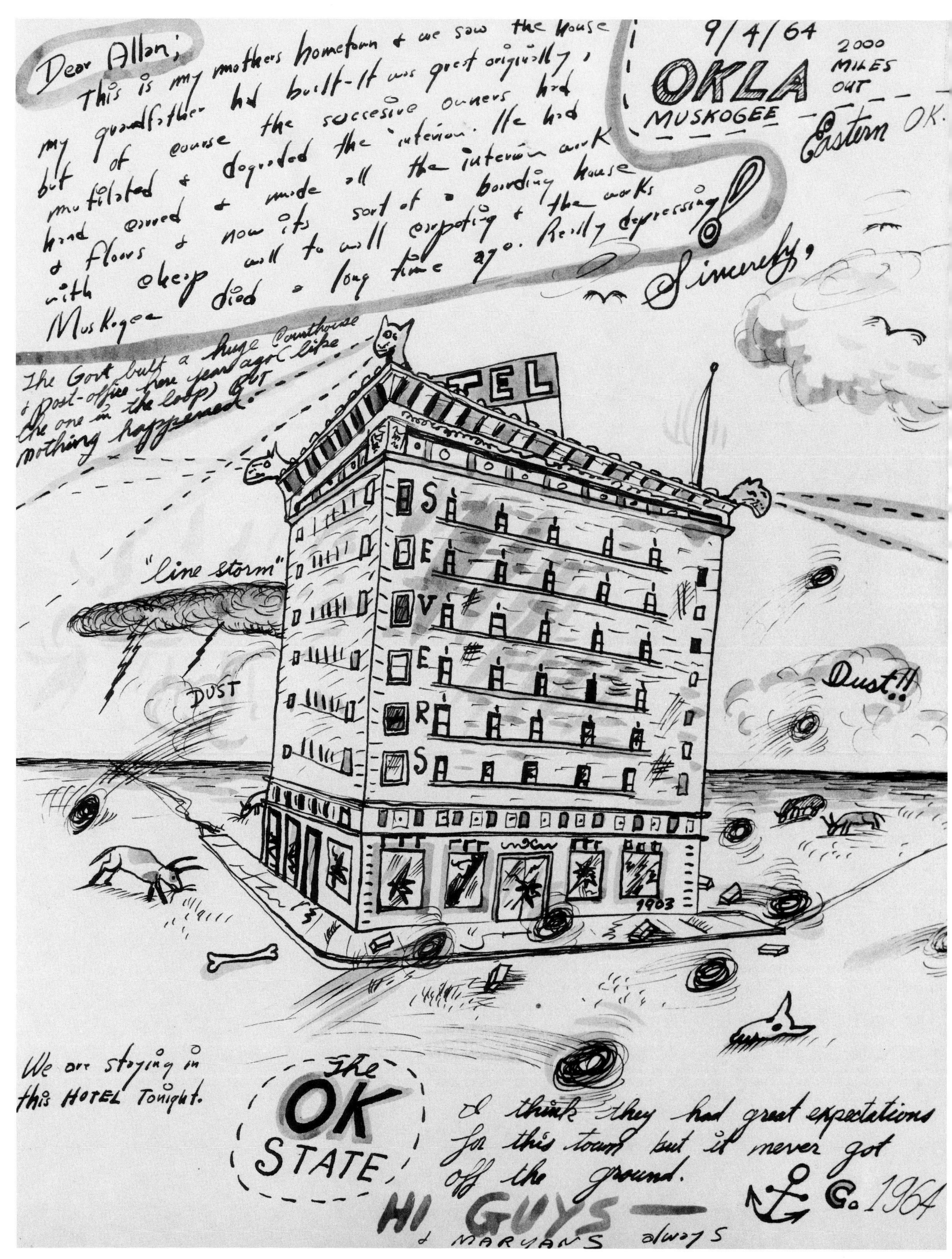

Dear Allan;
This is my mothers hometown & we saw the house my grandfather had built - It was great originally, but of course the successive owners had mutilated & degraded the interior. He had hand carved & made all the interior work & floors & now its sort of a boarding house with cheap wall to wall carpeting & the works. Really depressing!
Muskogee died a long time ago.
Sincerely,
9/4/64
OKLA
MUSKOGEE
2000 MILES OUT
Eastern OK.
The Govt built a huge Courthouse & post-office here years ago (like the one in the loop) but nothing happened.
TEL
S E V E R S
1903
"line storm"
DUST
Dust!!
We are staying in this HOTEL Tonight.
The OK STATE
I think they had great expectations for this town but it never got off the ground.
HI GUYS —
& MARYANNS always
© 1964

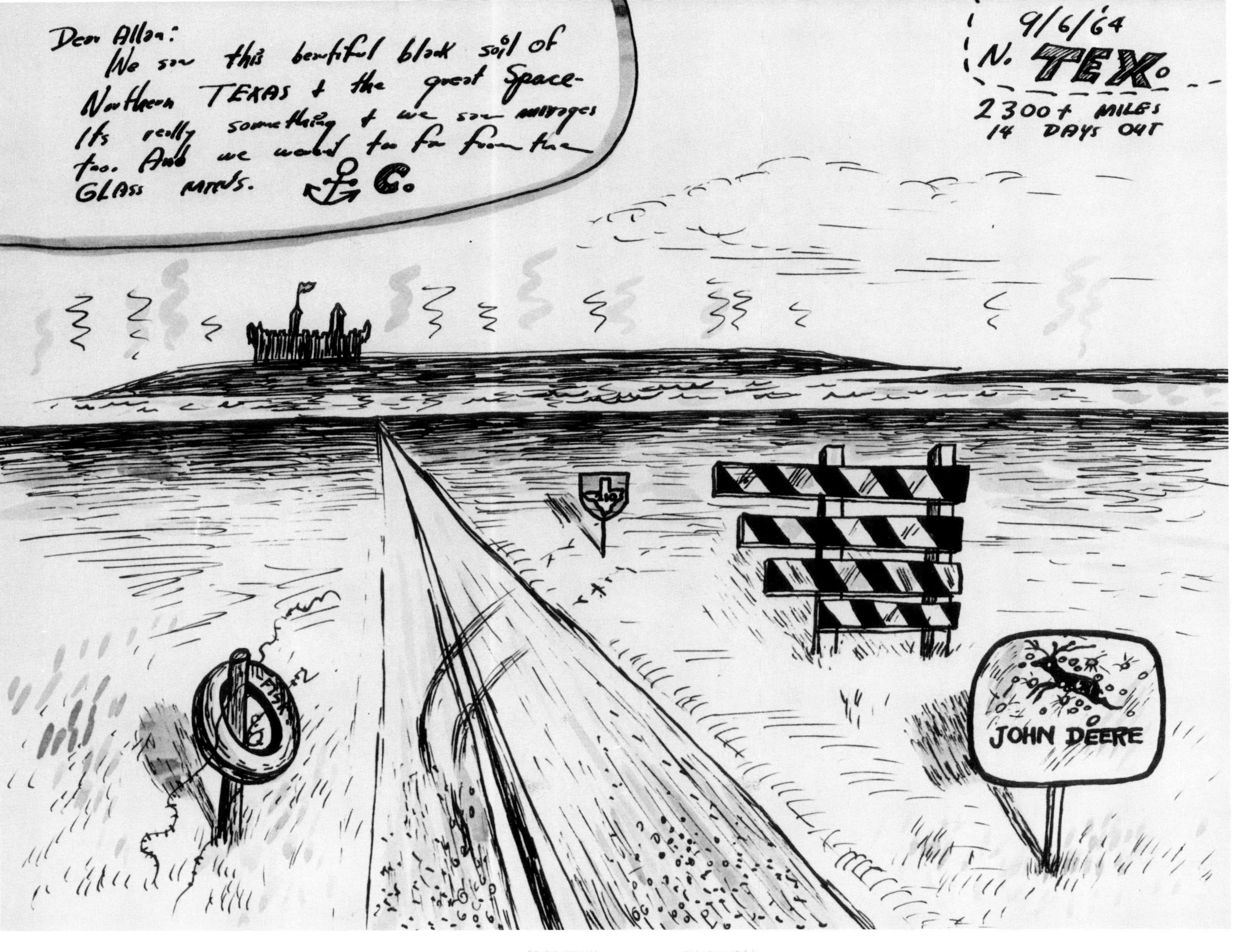
Dear Allan:
We saw this beautiful black soil of
Northern TEXAS + the great Space-
Its really something + we saw mirages
too. And we wanted too far from the
GLASS mirrors.
G.
9/6/64
N. TEX.
2300+ MILES
14 DAYS OUT
FISK
JOHN DEERE

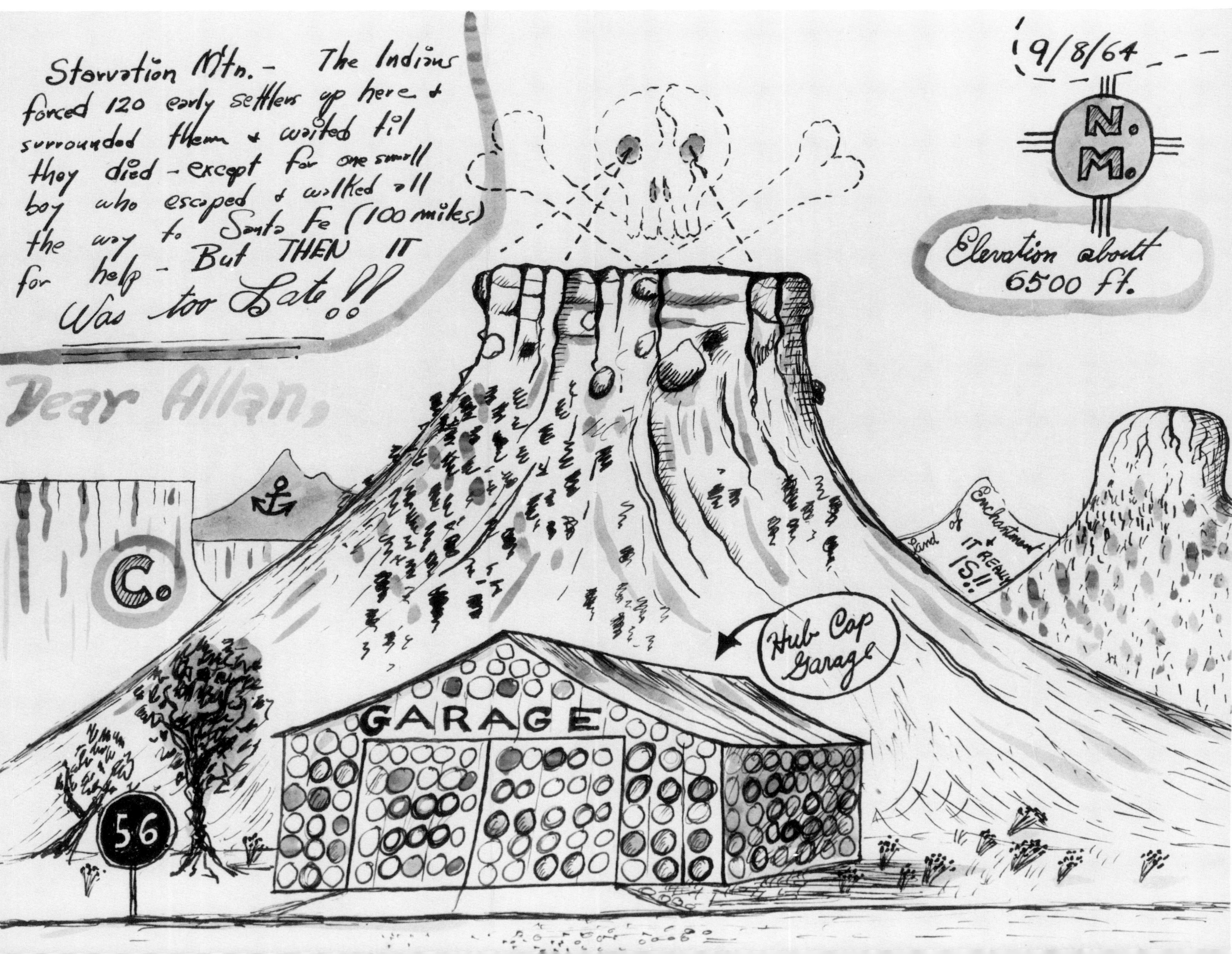

Starvation Mtn. – The Indians forced 120 early settlers up here & surrounded them & waited til they died – except for one small boy who escaped & walked all the way to Santa Fe (100 miles) for help – But THEN IT Was too Late!!
9/8/64
N. M.
Elevation about 6500 ft.
Dear Allan,
C.
Land of Enchantment & IT REALLY IS!!
Hub Cap Garage
GARAGE
56

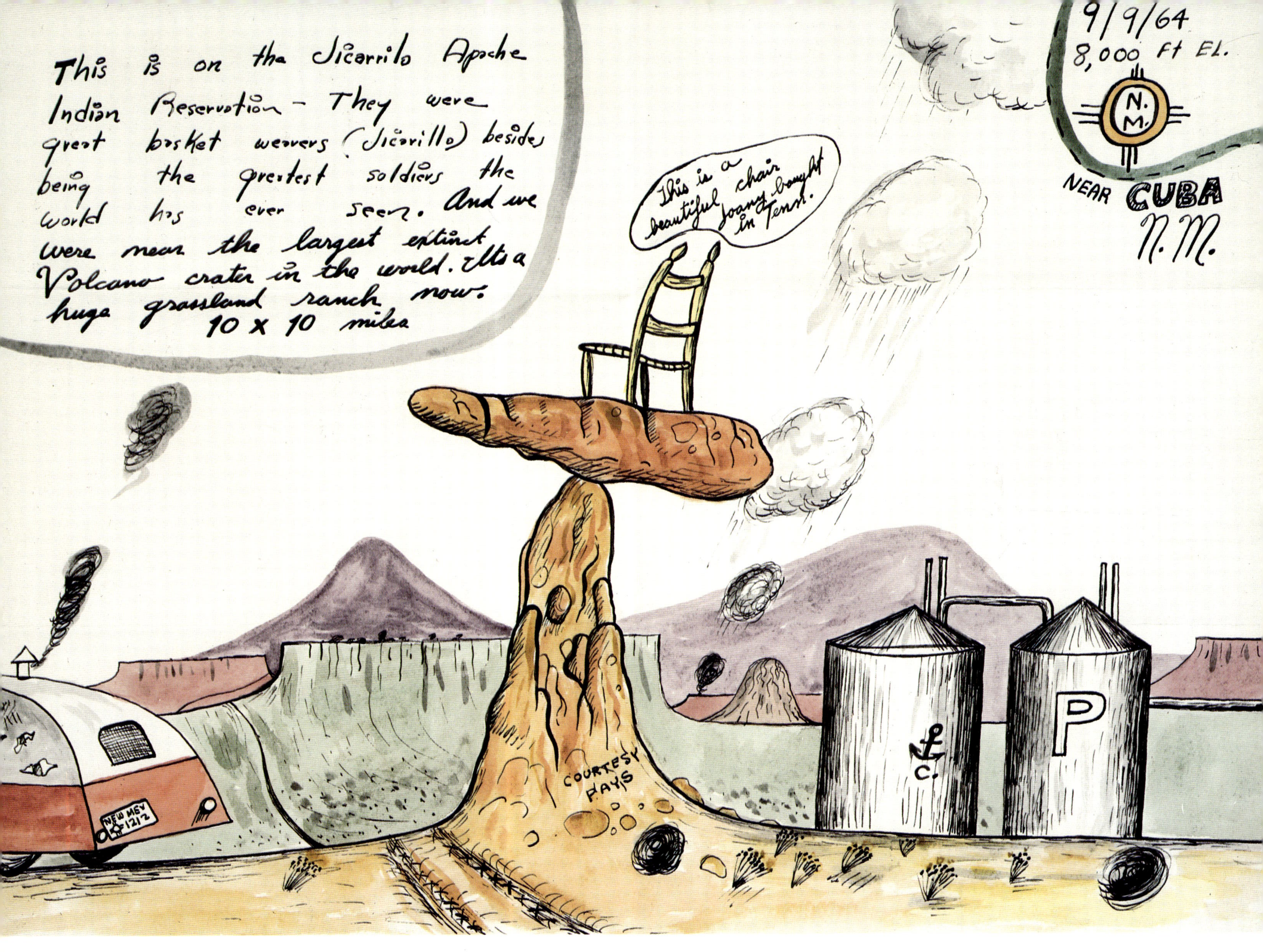
This is on the Jicarrilo Apache Indian Reservation - They were great basket weavers (Jicarillo) besides being the greatest soldiers the world has ever seen. And we were near the largest extinct Volcano crater in the world. Its a huge grassland ranch now. 10 x 10 miles
This is a beautiful chair Joany bought in Tenn.
9/9/64
8,000 Ft EL.
N. M.
NEAR CUBA
N. M.
COURTESY HAYS
P
C.
NEW MEX 1212

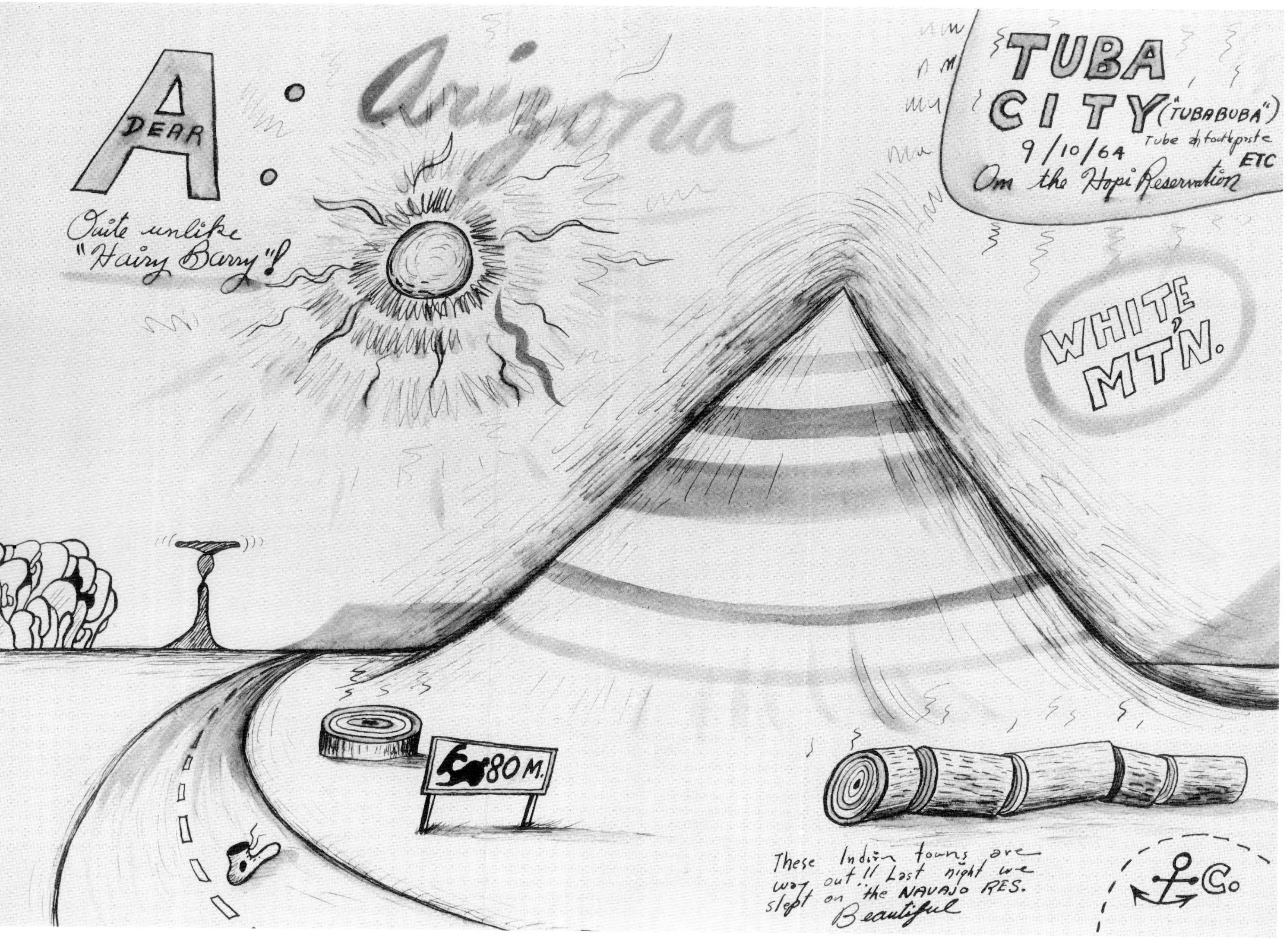

A
DEAR
A:
arizona
Quite unlike
"Hairy Barry"!
TUBA
CITY ("TUBABUBA")
9/10/64
ETC
On the Hopi Reservation
WHITE
MT'N.
80 M.
These Indian towns are
way out!! Last night we
slept on the NAVAJO RES.
Beautiful
Co

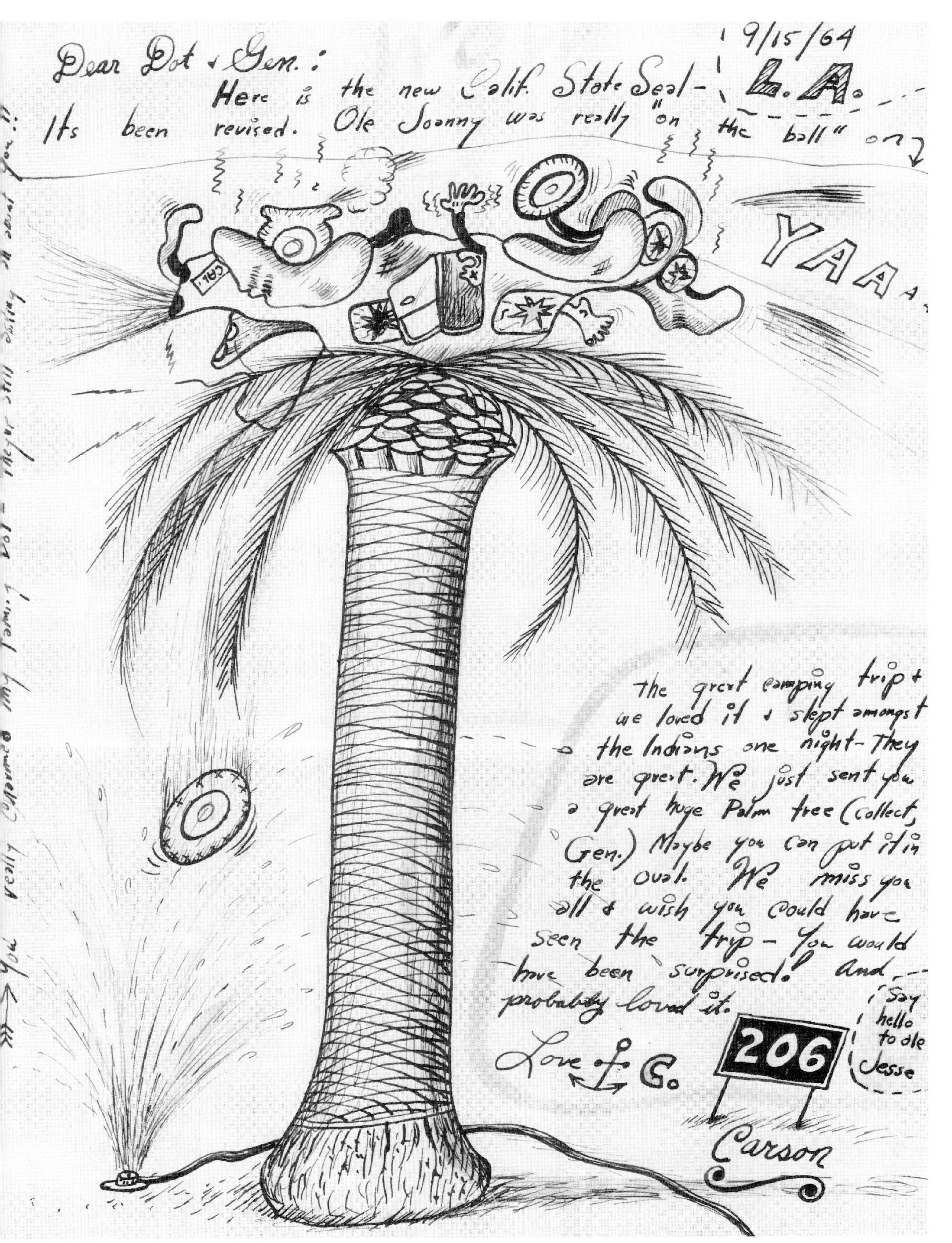

Dear Dot & Gen.:

9/15/64

L. A.

Here is the new Calif. State Seal - Its been revised. Ole Joanny was really "on the ball" on → you really charmed my family Dot - they're still asking me about you!!

The great camping trip & we loved it & slept amongst the Indians one night - They are great. We just sent you a great huge Palm tree (Collect, Gen.) Maybe you can put it in the Oval. We miss you all & wish you could have seen the trip - You would have been surprised! and probably loved it.

Love J & C.

Say hello to ole Jesse

Carson

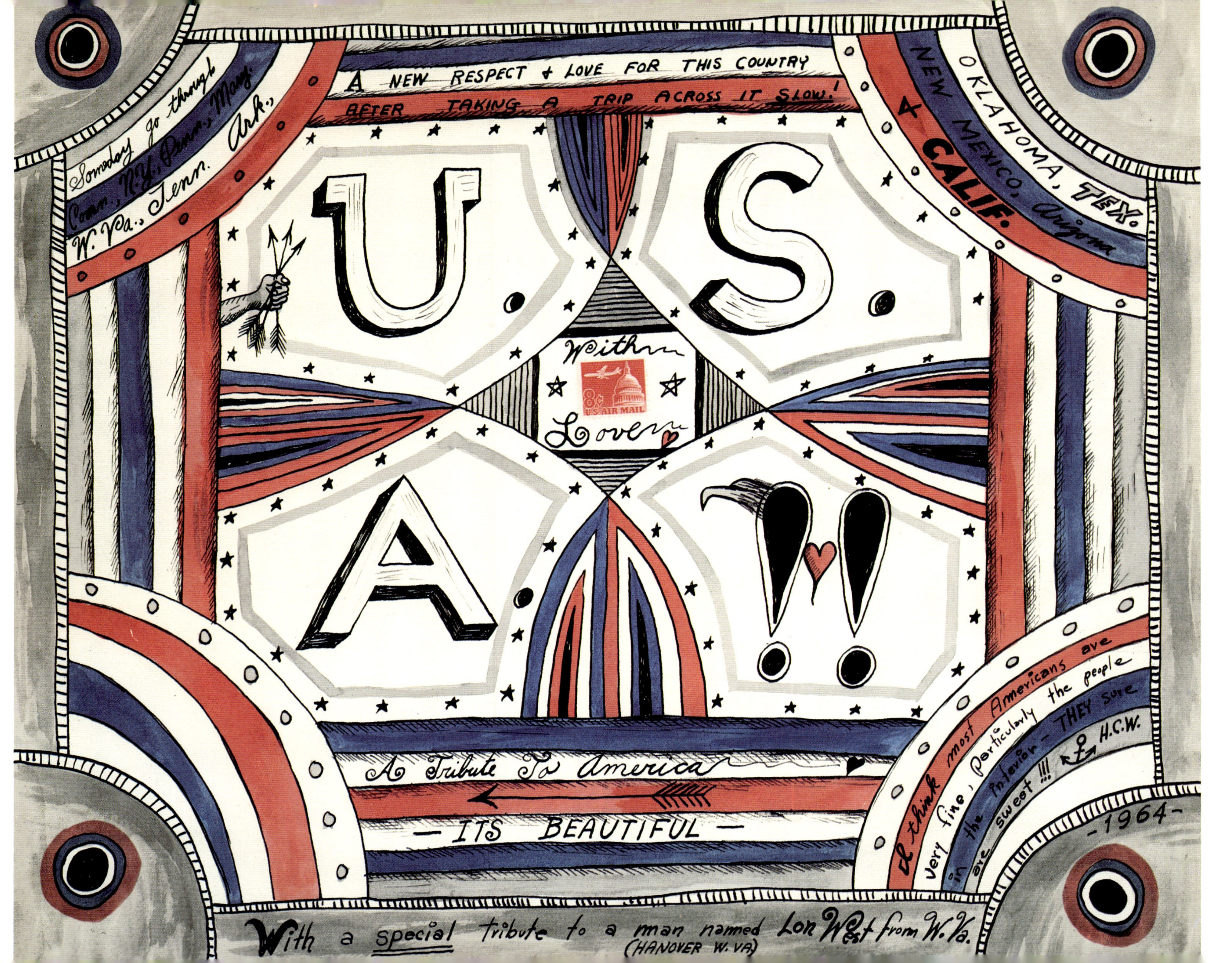
A NEW RESPECT + LOVE FOR THIS COUNTRY
AFTER TAKING A TRIP ACROSS IT SLOW!
Someday go through
Conn., N.Y., Penn., Mary.
W. Va., Tenn. Ark.,
OKLAHOMA, TEX.
NEW MEXICO, Arizona
+ CALIF.
U.S.A.!!
With Love
8¢ U.S. AIR MAIL
A Tribute To America
— ITS BEAUTIFUL —
I think most Americans are
very fine, particularly the people
in the interior – THEY sure
are sweet!!!
H.C.W.
-1964-
With a special tribute to a man named Lon West from W. Va.
(HANOVER W. VA)

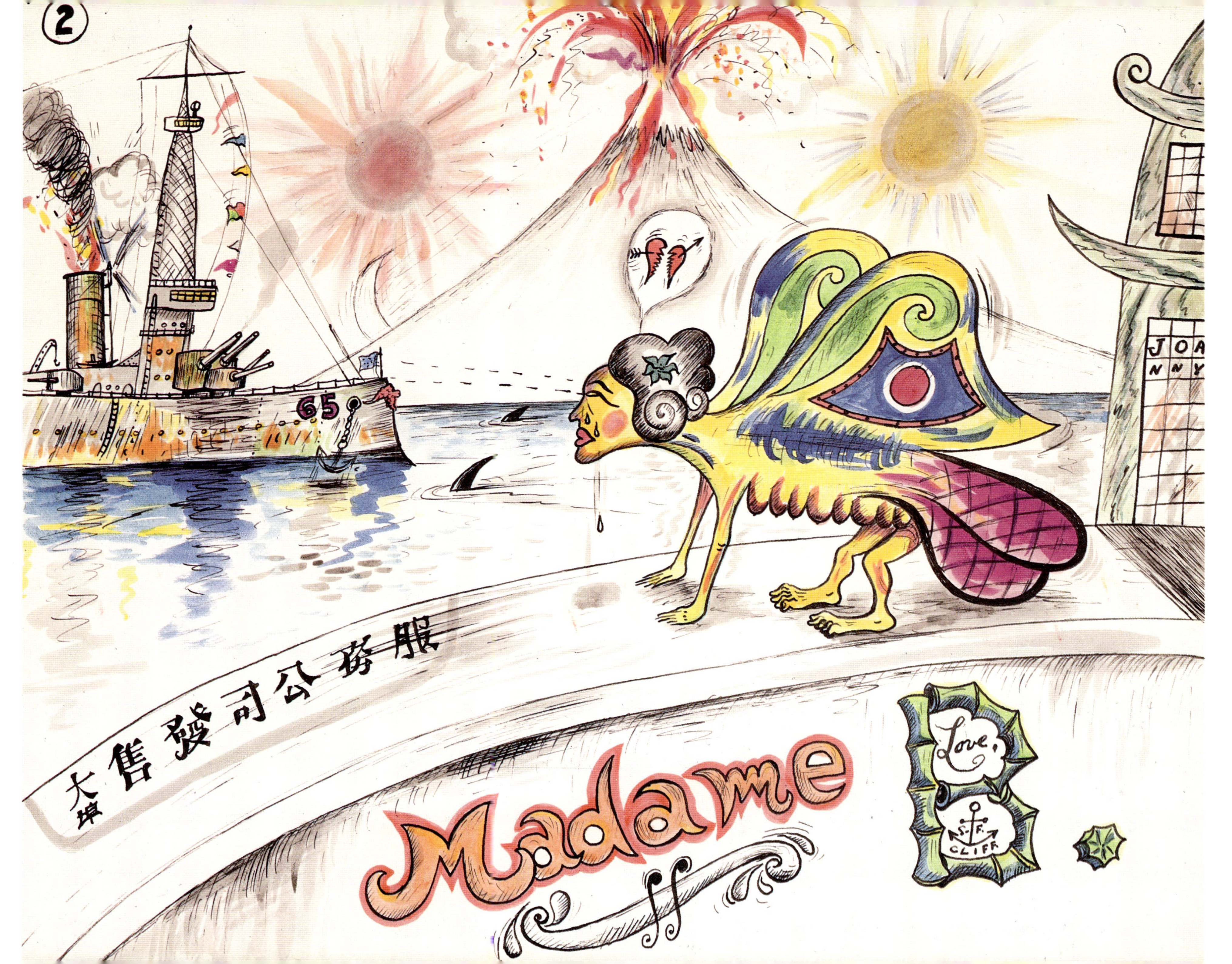
2
65
大埠售發司公務服
Madame B.
Love,
S.F.
CLIFF

Sculpture

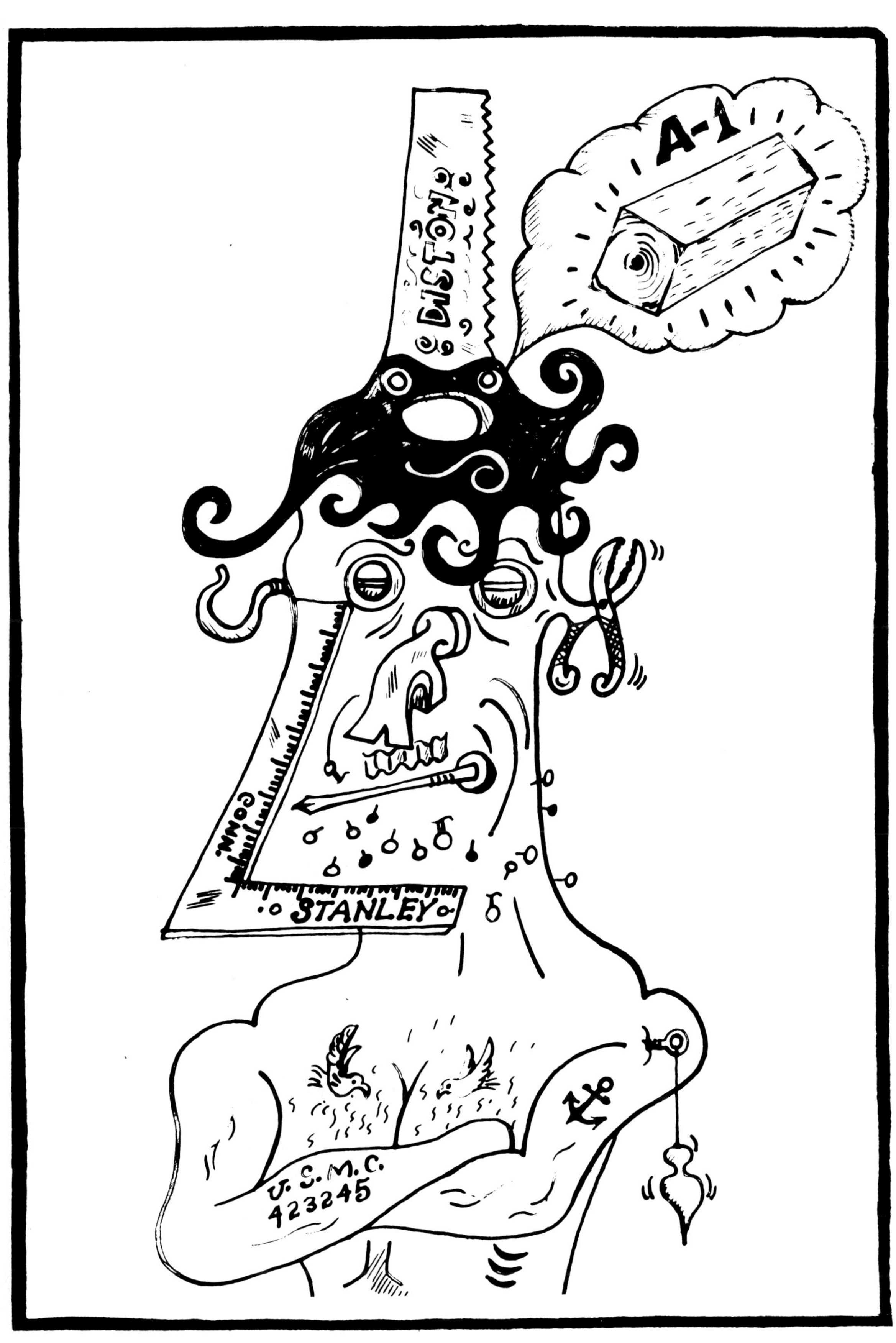

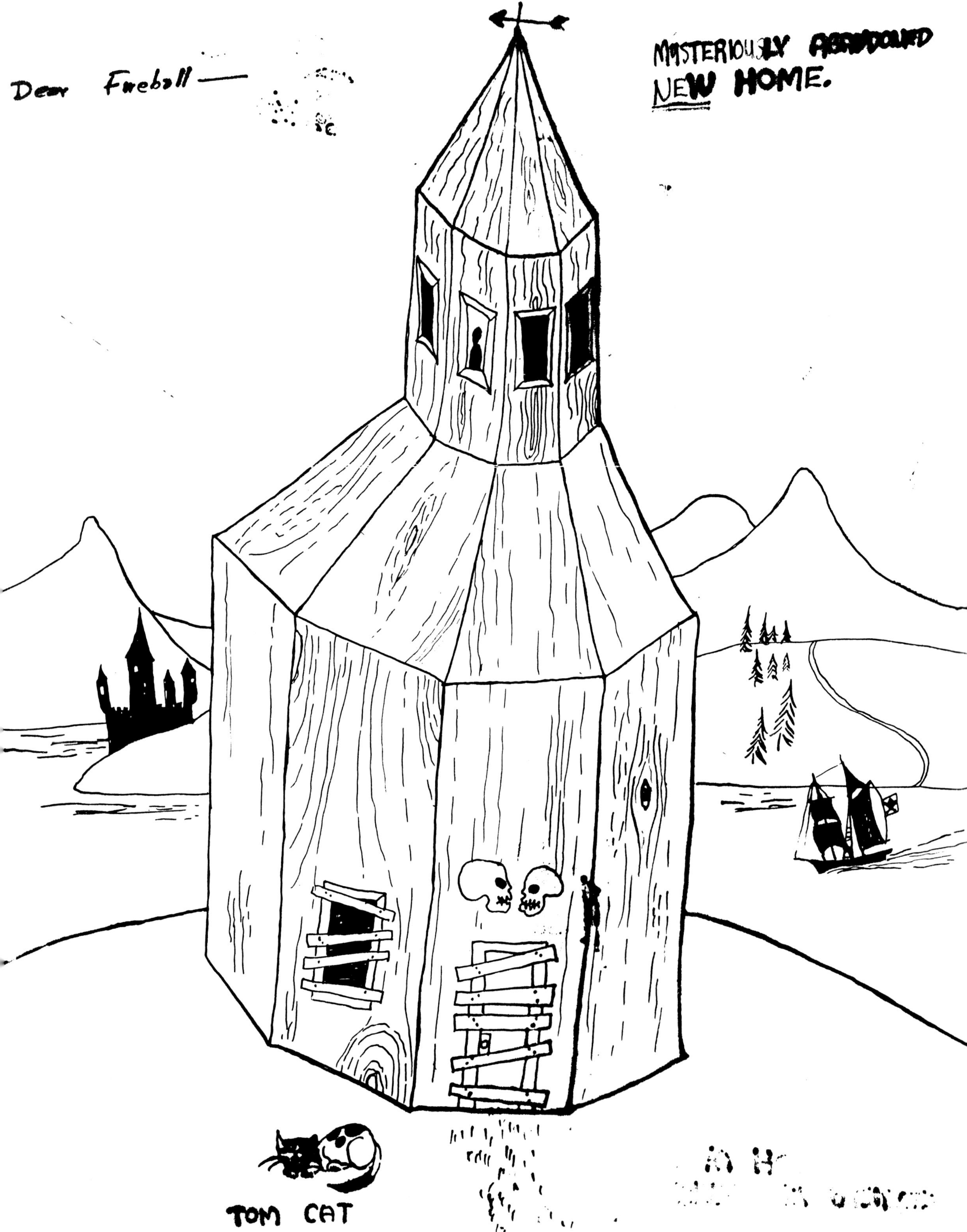
Dear Fireball —
MYSTERIOUSLY ABANDONED NEW HOME.
TOM CAT

from a letter to Martha and Mike Renner 1959

The show came off fine and I'm glad it's launched. Openings are sort of thrilling but it's always a terrible ordeal for me to meet lots of people. I'm not very sociable or verbal so its painful. I'm glad I don't have to suffer through these often. I just finished a new piece and it was such an emotional experience it made me deathly sick for a while. Finally after weeks of intense painful and exciting moments I realized it could never be lost (solved) and that I had it. — I just fell apart literally and was horrible sick and torn up. But this is what it takes and I'm glad to accept these challenges and try to do my best. I guess I've got a real demon in me and I'm glad. He can use me to death.

from a letter to Martha and Mike Renner February 27, 1964

Well I see some critic blasted my work again in the Pasadena show. Critics in general are rooted to the "European tradition" of art + can't seem to break with that. They are so conventional + nasty + invariably see the wrong things in a piece of art even when they praise it, which is seldom. Fortunately I do not make art for the critics, or anyone. I make them to please myself + never on the level of sheer entertainment. It goes much deeper than that.

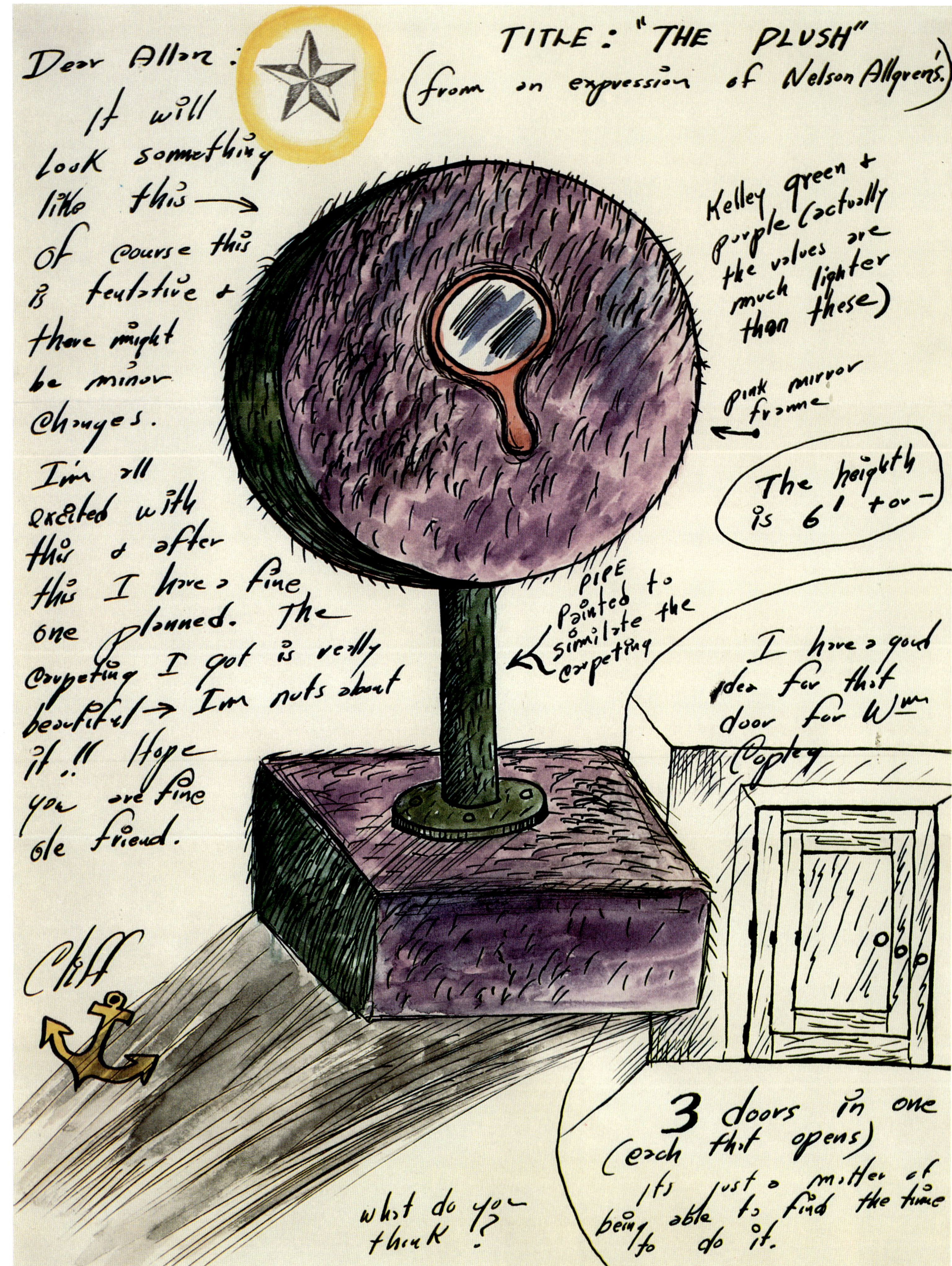
TITLE: "THE PLUSH"
(from an expression of Nelson Allgren's)
Dear Allan:
It will look something like this →
Of course this is tentative & there might be minor changes.
I'm all excited with this & after this I have a fine one planned. The carpeting I got is really beautiful → I'm nuts about it.!! Hope you are fine ole friend.
Clift
Kelley green & purple (actually the values are much lighter than these)
pink mirror frame
The heighth is 6' +or-
PIPE Painted to similate the carpeting
I have a good idea for that door for Wm Copley
3 doors in one (each that opens)
its just a matter of being able to find the time to do it.
what do you think?

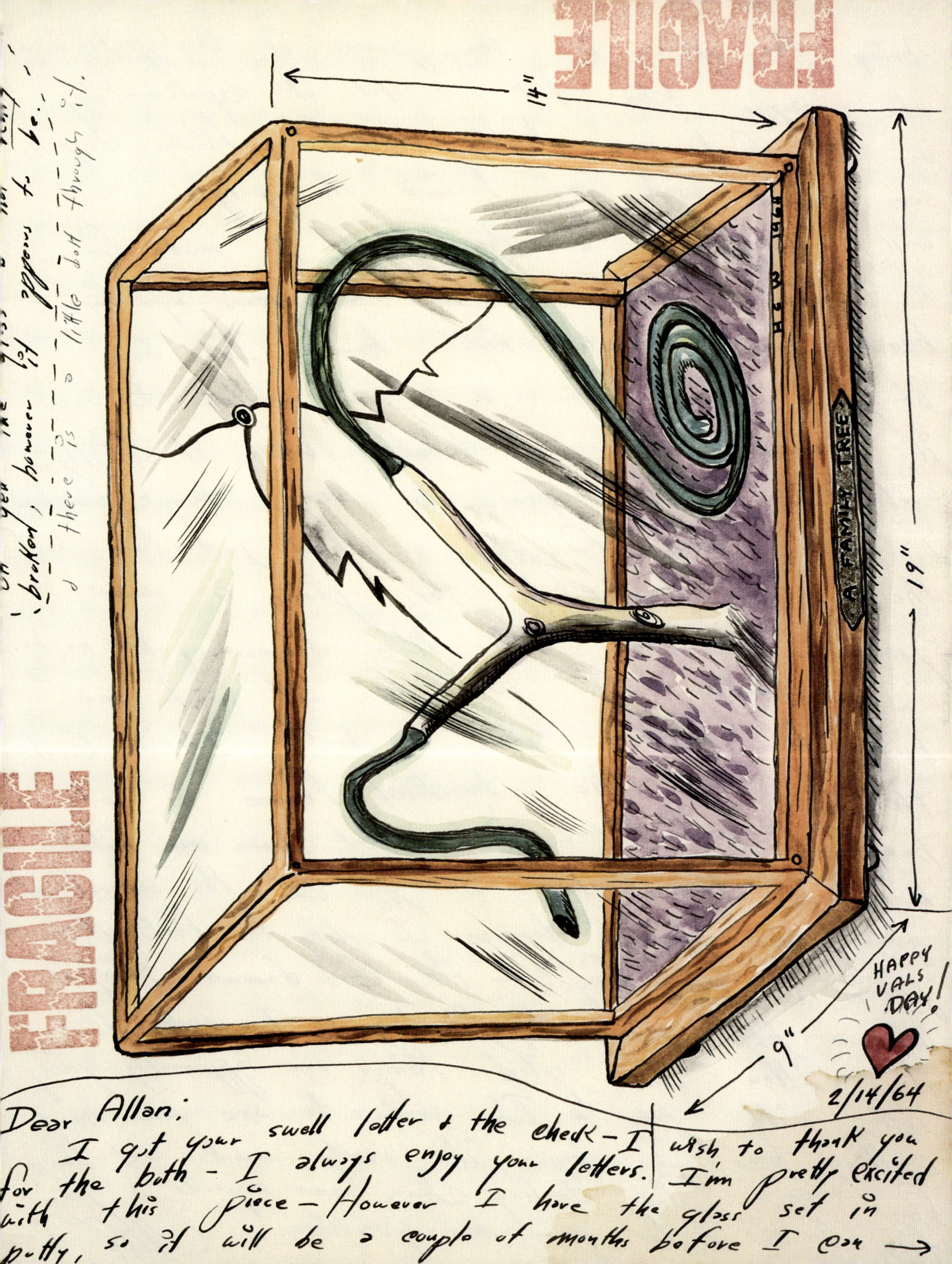

2/14/64

Dear Allan:
I got your swell letter & the check – I wish to thank you for the both – I always enjoy your letters. I'm pretty excited with this piece – However I have the glass set in putty, so it will be a couple of months before I can →

\#1

Dear Allan:

Douglas Fir 2/26/64

Actually the piece is more effective than this little drawing & the proportion of the piece is different. The lines of the falling form were ground in by hand with a carborundum stone & seem to work. I like the piece & feel I have extended my idea of the use of the mirrors. It's a small piece & I'm very excited with it & its finished now. (there is a very strange greenish caste to these mirrors somehow)

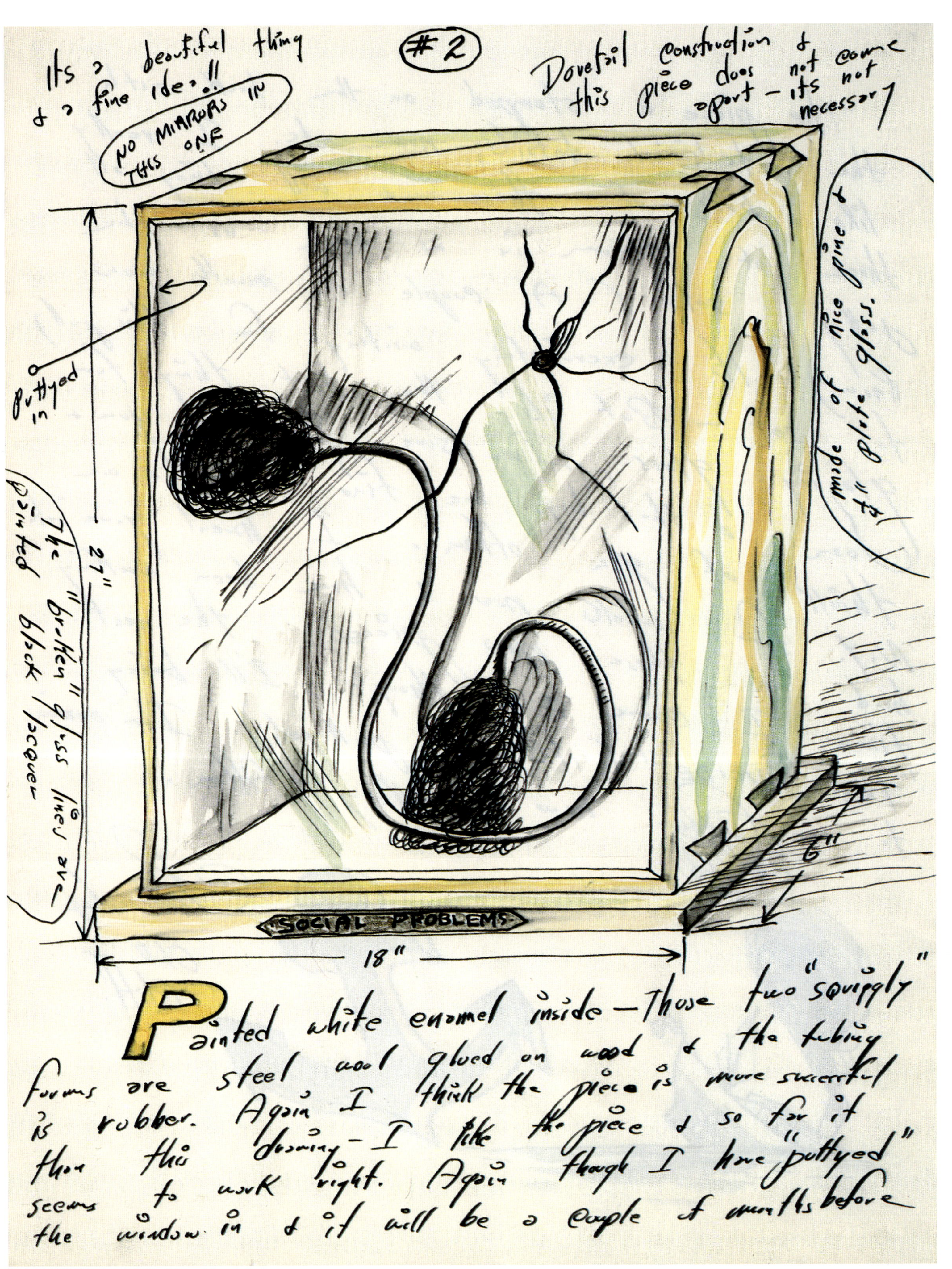

Its a beautiful thing & a fine idea!!
#2
Dovetail construction & this piece does not come apart - its not necessary
NO MIRRORS IN THIS ONE
made of nice pine & 1" plate glass.
puttyed in
The "broken" glass lines are painted black lacquer
27"
6"
SOCIAL PROBLEMS
18"
Painted white enamel inside — Those two "squiggly" forms are steel wool glued on wood & the tubing is rubber. Again I think the piece is more successful than this drawing — I like the piece & so far it seems to work right. Again though I have "puttyed" the window in & it will be a couple of months before

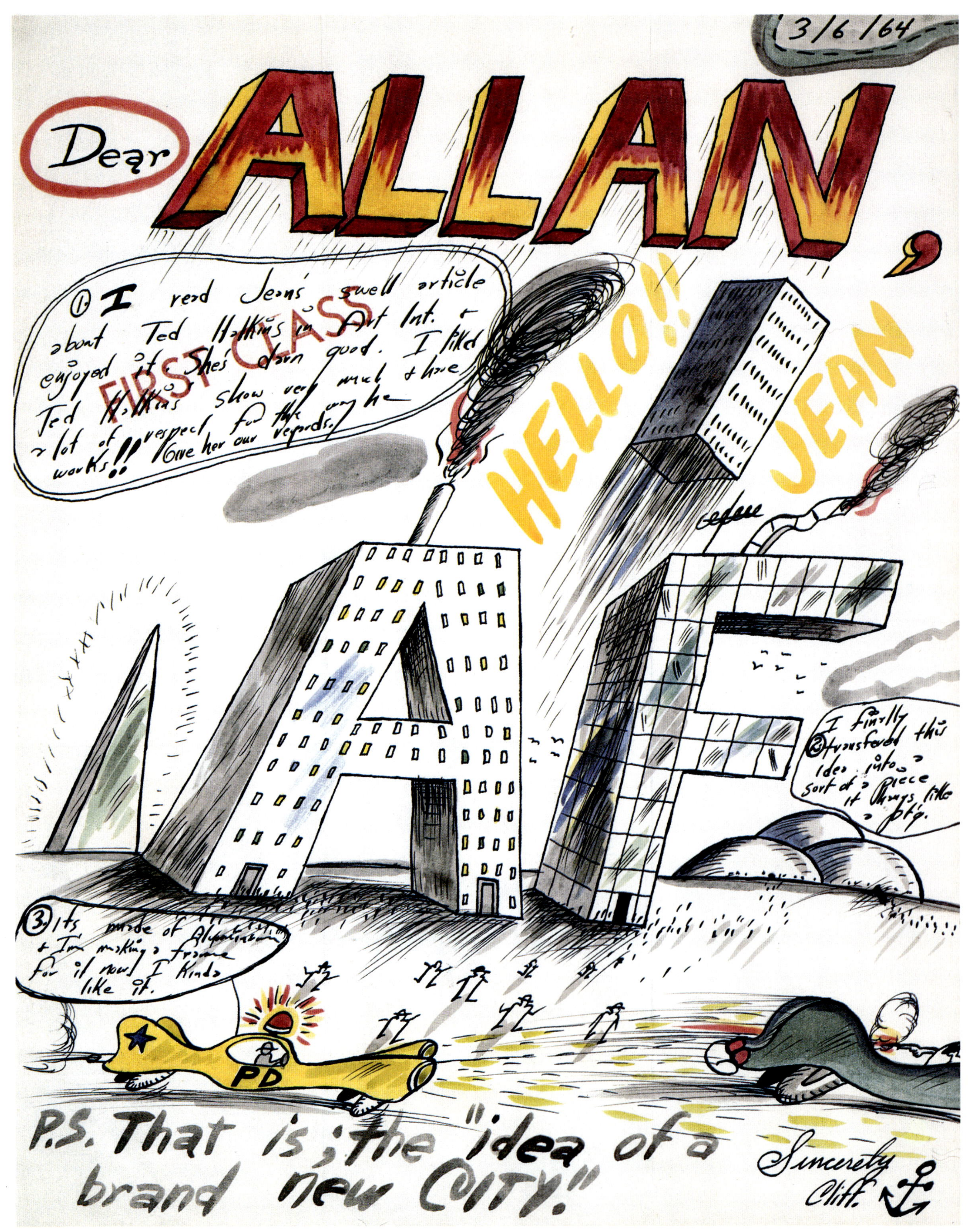
3/6/64
Dear ALLAN,
1. I read Jean's swell article about Ted Halkins in Art Int. & enjoyed it. She's darn good. I liked Ted Halkins show very much & have a lot of respect for the way he works!! Give her our regards.
FIRST CLASS
HELLO!! JEAN
I finally 2. transfered this idea into a sort of a piece it looks like a ptg.
3. Its made of Aluminium & Im making a frame for it now! I kinda like it.
PD
P.S. That is; the "idea of a brand new CITY."
Sincerely Cliff.

② Its more like this than the other drawing

THE BEGINNING OF A BRAND NEW CITY

1964

H.C. WESTERMANN

I haven't made the frame yet, so its tentative – I think it will be of pine though ??

made of 1/8" Aluminum bars & plate alum.

1/4" glass front over the Alum. drawing

mirror

The drawing is engraved into the Alum. & the lettering is stamped in with my steel letters.

These pieces of Alum are nailed on a piece of plywood

I think it looks very neat & clean without being slick.

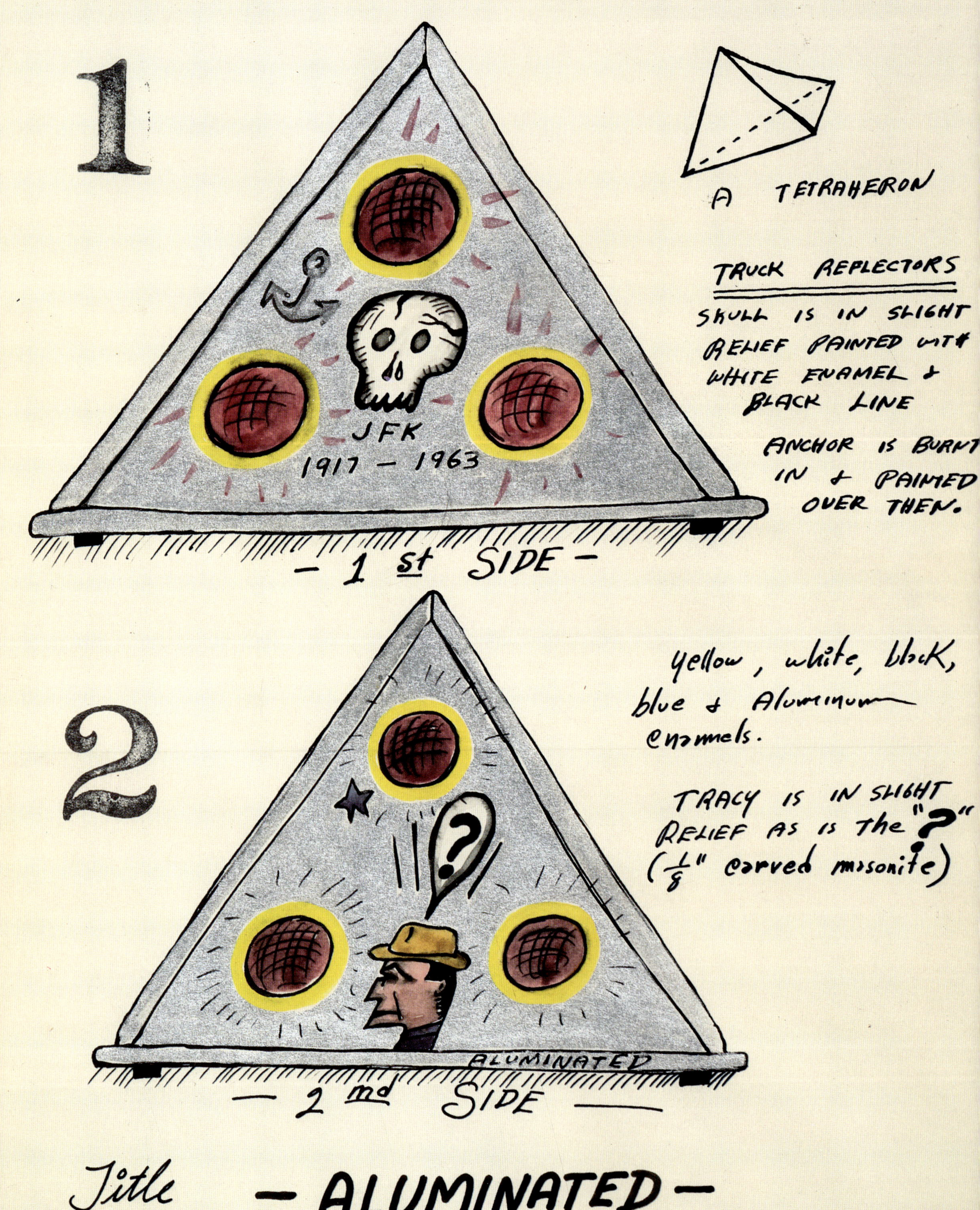
1
A TETRAHERON
TRUCK REFLECTORS
SKULL IS IN SLIGHT RELIEF PAINTED WITH WHITE ENAMEL & BLACK LINE
ANCHOR IS BURNT IN & PAINTED OVER THEN.
JFK
1917 – 1963
– 1 st SIDE –
2
yellow, white, black, blue & Aluminum enamels.
TRACY IS IN SLIGHT RELIEF AS IS THE "?" (1/8" carved masonite)
?
ALUMINATED
– 2 nd SIDE –
Title – ALUMINATED –
(I think its beautiful)

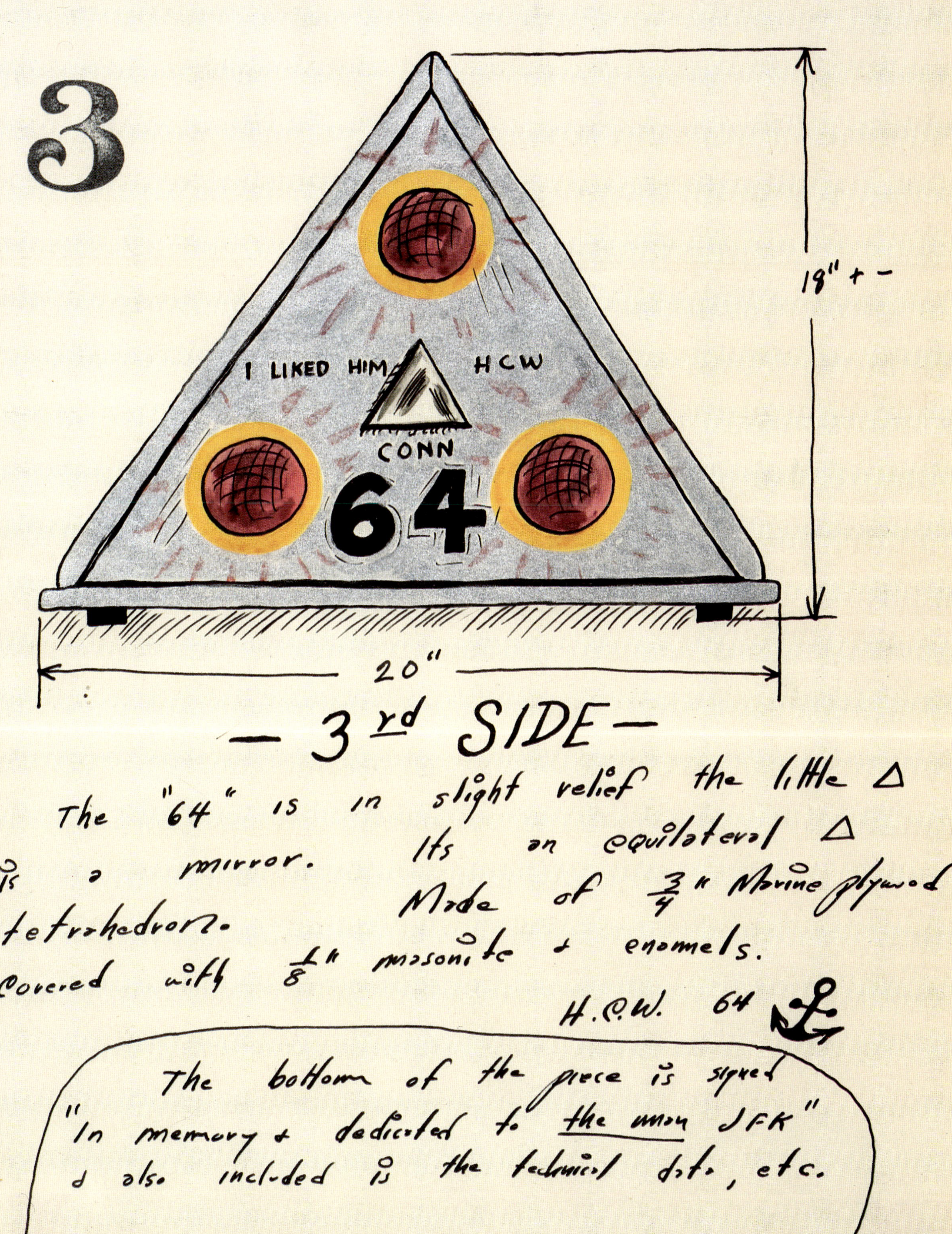
3
I LIKED HIM
HCW
CONN
64
18" + -
20"
— 3rd SIDE —
The "64" is in slight relief the little △
is a mirror. Its an equilateral △
tetrahedron. Made of 3/4" Marine plywood
Covered with 1/8" masonite & enamels.
H.C.W. 64
The bottom of the piece is signed
"In memory & dedicated to the man JFK"
& also included is the technical data, etc.

February 17, 1965

Dear Allan:

I received your good letter + appreciate your writing. I'm glad things are going well & Maryan's show is underway. I'd like to see it. He's a real fine artist. I sure like him & his wife. They have been very nice to us. I don't think I ever thanked you for January's check. I did receive this month's check too + wish to thank you for both of them. And appreciate you trying to get them here earlier. I know you're constantly harassed & ole Cliff doesn't like to add to it, Allan, + hound you. I really hate that. I know you try your damndest. I'll let you be the judge on sending these new ones to England — You know what you're doing. However:
#1 — I don't like England (or France) in relationship to Art, etc.
#2 — By the time you get these back they will be beat up + dirty + of course they won't all be there (they should all be shown together, as they are closely related + each is an outgrowth of the proceeding one. For instance all the round ones are suns, of a sort I think — & one missing from the group wouldn't be right.
#3 — I am an American artist + don't give one God damn about the international scene (which is pretty weak in general).
#4 — I think this direction + form I am following is a good one + I believe it's honest. By the time, when + if you showed these, I think other artists in N.Y. would be trying the same. You know how many N.Y. artists imitate a form or technique etc. + steal from others no matter whether it's good or bad. Let's face it.

I have a lot of pride in my work — it's not like the other artists' work + I don't want it to be. I want it to be mine (or something of the spirit, maybe something a hell of a lot better + of a higher order than me). I don't think I'm precious or that my work is "above" showing in England — that's not the point. Or whether I like England or France or Switzerland (they did make the cuckoo clock though).

Now you mentioned what happens in the next couple of months. (Oh yeh when I say my work is not like the other artists — I don't mean to intimidate their efforts, as there are a lot of very fine "other" artists). Well now I think the way these are developing + they are "swinging" I think I am good for four or five more months of these. I'm just coming into my own now + am really excited with them + they are larger now. These last two are 20″ × 30″ solid mahogany pieces (not glued up either) + they are beautiful. It's next to impossible to draw these as the reliefs look + have an entirely different feeling. Now supposing I sent these 12 reliefs off to England — It would be like starting again. I need the ones I've done to study (very important) + the more I have the more good I get out of studying them. I know this must be hard for you to understand.

These things are very introspective + meditative + the thought of splitting them up until I am finished with this series is very revolting. As a consequence each new one is really a revelation + exciting. For instance I've been studying #1, #2, + #3 + it's helped me with #11. You see I learn from my own efforts + not somebody else's. Even the size is related to the proceeding one. I'm not saying if you sell these they should all go together — that's not it (however one is a triptych).

And I do not want to have to work on these with the idea of "hurry, hurry, hurry, remember the London show." I have been working long + hard but it's been exciting + not under pressure. Well ole Allan I'm an odd duck aren't I? But I do love you guys anyway + I'm not trying to tell you what to do. I sure love ole Dennis!

Sincerely, Cliff

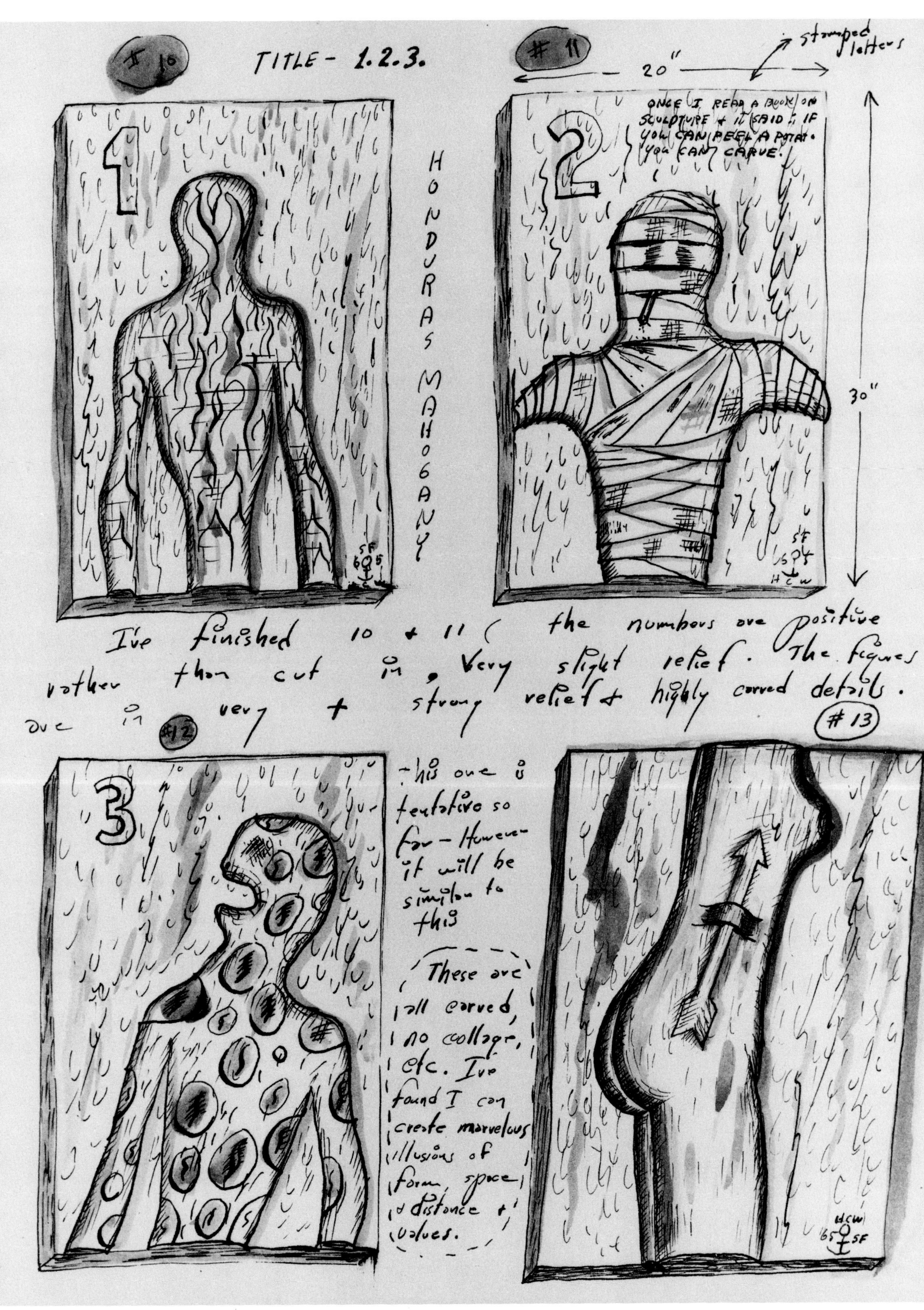

10
TITLE - 1.2.3.
11
20"
stamped letters
ONCE I READ A BOOK ON SCULPTURE + IT SAID : IF YOU CAN PEEL A POTATO YOU CAN CARVE.
1
HONDURAS MAHOGANY
2
30"
I've finished 10 + 11 (the numbers are positive rather than cut in, very slight relief. The figures are in very + strong relief + highly carved details.
#12
#13
3
this one is tentative so far - However it will be similar to this
These are all carved, no collage, etc. I've found I can create marvelous illusions of form, space + distance + values.

3/5/65

Dear Allan:

This is the 14th one + is carved out of a solid piece of Hon. Mahogany 20x20 + 1" thick – The title is: "Manifesto of the GREAT SOCIETY": it turned out real good + the carving is really swinging now. Oh yeh I heard that "music" Allan!

The last one: "The woman from Angel Island", you know, the one with the arrow, is finished too.

I've found that carving does not have to be carving in the conventional sense + I can see it is an completely unlimited technique or direction, as you wish – The real possibilities have only been scratched at. These have been exciting ones + of course the later ones are a better expression than the early ones (mine I mean)

I failed to mention that I made two small pieces (3 dimension) as I did these carvings: one is a teak wood ship (an extension of those I did in Chicago + its a good one.

I don't know how this came about after so many years, but I had this strong desire to do it. And the other one is called "THE SLOB"— The colors of this piece are beautiful & the piece seems to work - I've been studying it off and on for weeks now. I am going to let the carvings go for a while now & do two fairly large pieces (in the round) that I have been planning & am ready to go on. It seems that the grocery store next door discards wooden boxes every day (good ones) & I have been trying to figure, ever since we came, what I could use them for — Finally I got it & hence they will be used in one of these two pieces (hundreds of them) Its a fantastic idea & the piece will take weeks to make. Well Allan ole friend — I realize this is strickly an "I", "I", "I" letter & I apologize - However I've never been so excited working - Things are "jelling" now. Tell Dennis we sure loved his fine letter & say hello to Frankie boy.

Say Hello to Jean!

Cliff

REAL HAMMER - A "CHEAP" ONE

22"

SOLID ALUMINUM (The metal not that god damned "sculp-metal")

THE SLOB

WESTERMANN

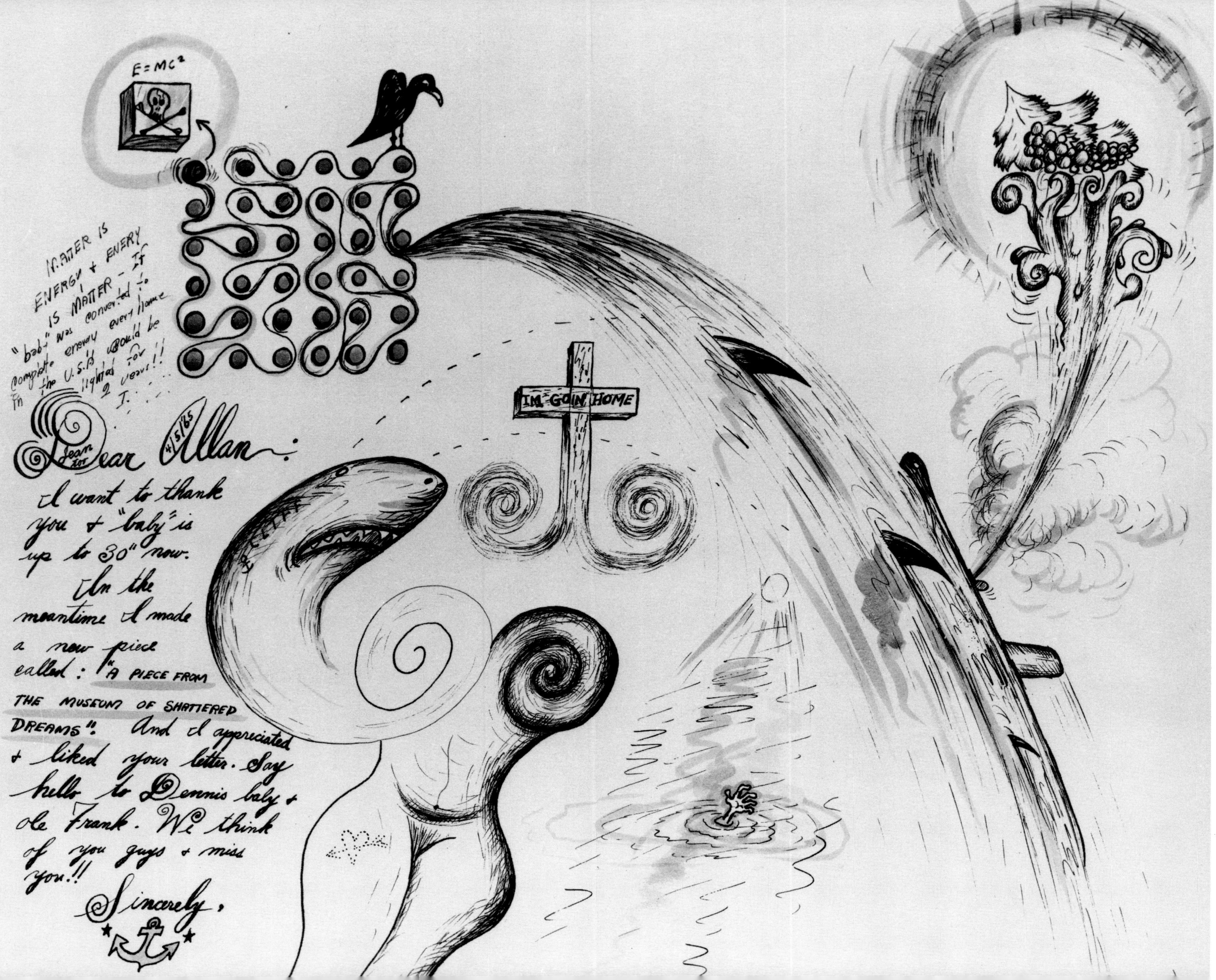

4/5/65

Dear Allan:

I want to thank you + "baby" is up to 30" now.

In the meantime I made a new piece called: "A PIECE FROM THE MUSEUM OF SHATTERED DREAMS". And I appreciated + liked your letter. Say hello to Dennis baby + ole Frank. We think of you guys + miss you!!

Sincerely,

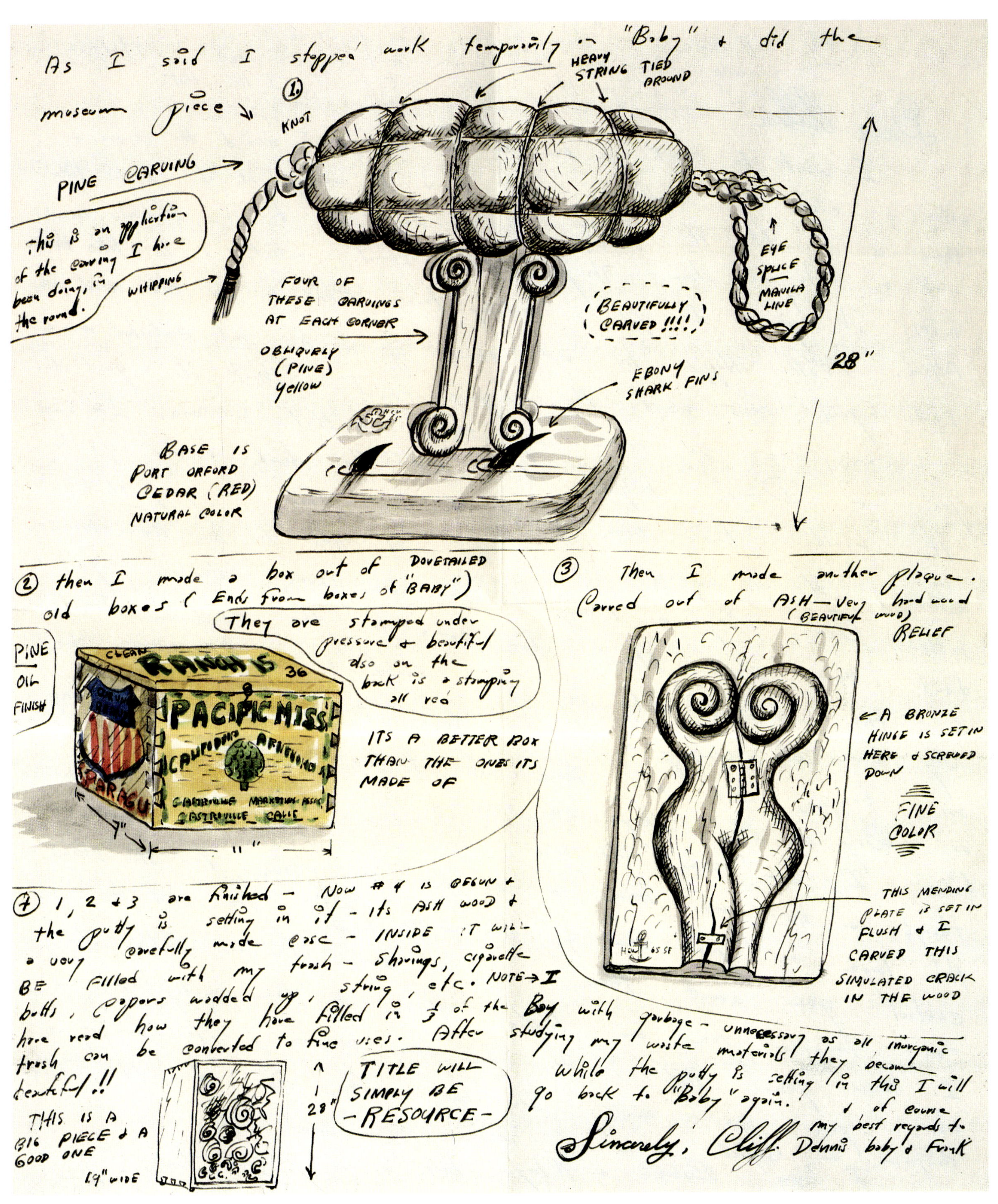

As I said I stopped work temporarily on "Baby" & did the museum piece →

1. HEAVY STRING TIED AROUND

KNOT

PINE CARVING →

this is an application of the carving I have been doing, in the round.

WHIPPING

FOUR OF THESE CARVINGS AT EACH CORNER →

OBLIQUELY (PINE) yellow

BEAUTIFULLY CARVED !!!!

EYE SPLICE MANILA LINE

28"

EBONY SHARK FINS

BASE IS PORT ORFORD CEDAR (RED) NATURAL COLOR

2. then I made a box out of DOVETAILED old boxes (Ends from boxes of "BABY")

They are stamped under pressure & beautiful also on the back is a stamping all red

PINE OIL FINISH

CLEAN RANCH'S 36 PACIFIC MISS CALIFORNIA ARTICHOKES CALIFORNIA MARKETING ASSOC CASTROVILLE CALIF PARAGU

7" 11"

ITS A BETTER BOX THAN THE ONES ITS MADE OF

3. Then I made another plaque. Carved out of ASH — very hard wood (BEAUTIFUL wood) RELIEF

← A BRONZE HINGE IS SET IN HERE & SCREWED DOWN

FINE COLOR

THIS MENDING PLATE IS SET IN FLUSH & I CARVED THIS SIMULATED CRACK IN THE WOOD

HCW 65 SF

4. 1, 2 & 3 are finished — Now # 4 is BEGUN & the putty is setting in it — its ASH wood & a very carefully made case — INSIDE IT WILL BE filled with my trash — shavings, cigarette butts, papers wadded up, string, etc. NOTE → I have read how they have filled in 1/3 of the Bay with garbage — unnecessary as all inorganic trash can be converted to fine uses. After studying my waste materials they become beautiful!!

THIS IS A BIG PIECE & A GOOD ONE

19" WIDE

28"

TITLE WILL SIMPLY BE — RESOURCE —

While the putty is setting in this I will go back to "Baby" again.

Sincerely, Cliff. & of course my best regards to Dennis baby & Frank

6/1/65

S.F.

Dear Allan:

Hope you are enjoying the country now - I'll bet its beautiful there. I hope that nice area never changes, as I remember it. As you know S.F. has been bombed + is a blight area - Completely poverty stricken, oh not in terms of $ + ¢, but really poverty stricken - There are 1,000,000 critics here + very few artists. The critics have ruined the city - For good!! So ole Joanny + I are moving on. We are going back to Conn. at Joannys' folks. We intend to go in July. I've still two more pieces to make, then we go. I've been working very hard + have made two more pieces since I wrote you last. I think you will be surprised with both of them - I really "went for it" + Boy oh Boy, they really feel good. They are both quite simple actually, but both ideas I am quite proud of! Brian O'D*** once wrote a review (he is a "CRITIC") to the effect the pieces were jokes. He should know I am deadly serious + have never made a "joke"

②

yet - For instance the "Walnut Box" was quite removed from being a mere joke - That box came right from my guts as have the ones I've done here. I wonder if he has ever gone into a gallery + picked up a piece + looked at the bottom of it or bothered to walk around behind a piece + study it. When I make a mockery or joke out of work - I will gladly sacrifice my other "ball" first. And I've only got one left. You know that operation etc. Ha, ha, ha. But then how many balls does a man need? Oh to hell with it.

① Carved out of a beautiful piece of maple - A very strange piece - I think its quite elegant! very structural too

handles are made of the same piece of maple + set + glued into a rabbett

4"

4"

NOWHERE

S.G. G.S.

H.C. ...

28"

(over →)

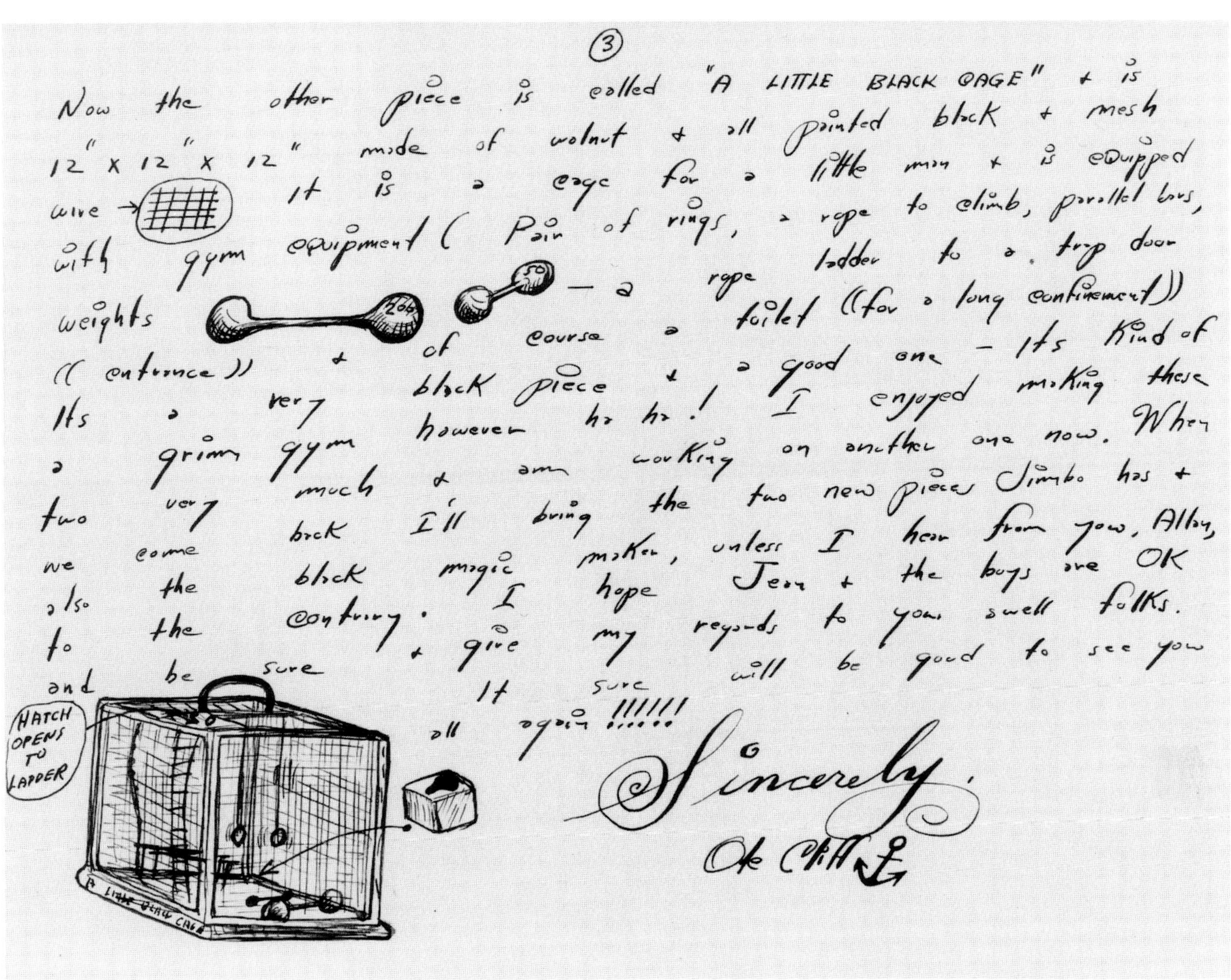
(3)

Now the other piece is called "A LITTLE BLACK CAGE" + is 12" x 12" x 12" made of walnut + all painted black + mesh wire → It is a cage for a little man + is equipped with gym equipment (Pair of rings, a rope to climb, parallel bars, weights — a rope ladder to a trap door ((entrance)) + of course a toilet ((for a long confinement)) Its a very black piece + a good one – Its kind of a grim gym however ha ha! I enjoyed making these two very much + am working on another one now. When we come back I'll bring the two new pieces Jimbo has + also the black magic maker, unless I hear from you. Alloy, to the contrary. I hope Jean + the boys are OK and be sure + give my regards to you swell folks. It sure will be good to see you all again!!!!!!......

Sincerely,

Ole Cliff

from a letter to Barbara Haskell October 30, 1977

You asked about "the Little Black Cage." Well I made that one in Frisco in '64 (I think) + it was an odd sort of thing. I had a real good feeling about the piece then + now + always wished, sort of, that I could see it again. It had strange things connected with it. It was a sort of miniature gymnasium with a little set of bar-bells + other related equipment + it was enclosed in this sort of animal cage. It was a nutty thing but when I made it it gave me a thrill, oh not because of the beauty of the thing so much as to the actual experience of building it. It was tiny, about 10" square as I remember. It was a miniature something or other + really the subject matter was not so important as the sheer feeling of making it at the fucking time + the place + the circumstances. I would not think of making that piece now of course. Oh my God what a long terrible description of a thing.

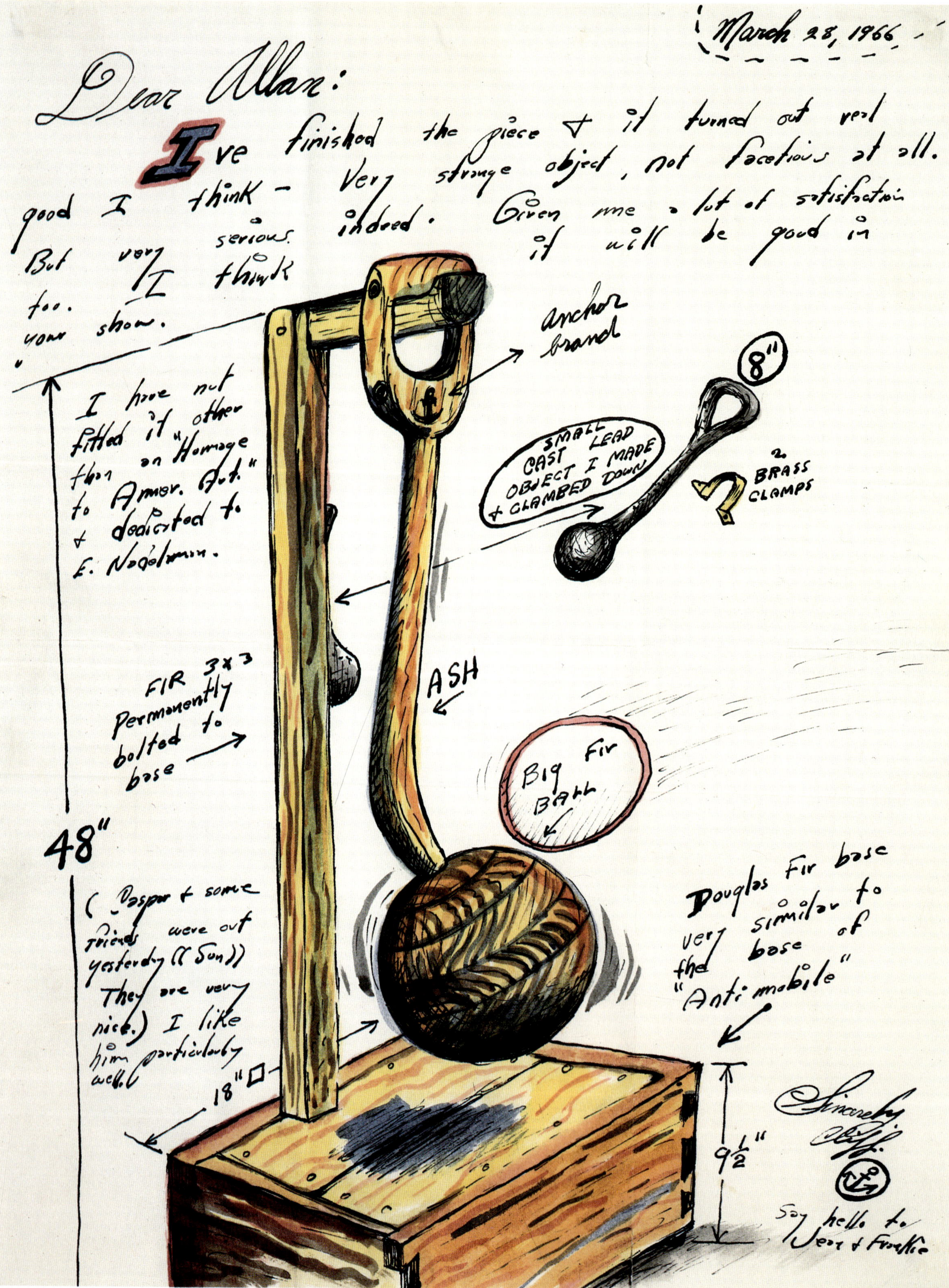

March 28, 1966

Dear Allan:

I've finished the piece & it turned out real good I think - Very strange object, not facetious at all. But very serious indeed. Given me a lot of satisfaction too. I think it will be good in your show.

anchor brand

8"

SMALL CAST LEAD OBJECT I MADE + CLAMBED DOWN

2 BRASS CLAMPS

I have not fitted it other than on "Homage to Amer. Art." & dedicated to E. Nadelman.

FIR 3x3 Permanently bolted to base

ASH

Big Fir BALL

48"

(Jasper & some friends were out yesterday ((Sun)) They are very nice.) I like him particularly well.

18" □

Douglas Fir base very similar to the base of "Anti mobile"

9½"

Sincerely
Cliff.

Say hello to Jean & Frankie

7/27/66

Dear Allen:

I finished the piece & like it very much. I used J. dodd car tires as a giant stamp pad & they worked fine. The ship is a good one, strange & beautiful. I fondled this ship 10,000 times before I glassed it in. (I really did drive right over the ship on the interesting technique)

DEATH SHIP — RUNOVER — BY A '66 LINCOLN CONTINENTAL

ON A SEA OF 1 $ BILLS.

PIECE IS 12" x 30".

PINE CONSTRUCTION & 1/4" plate glass windows puttied.

Cliff.

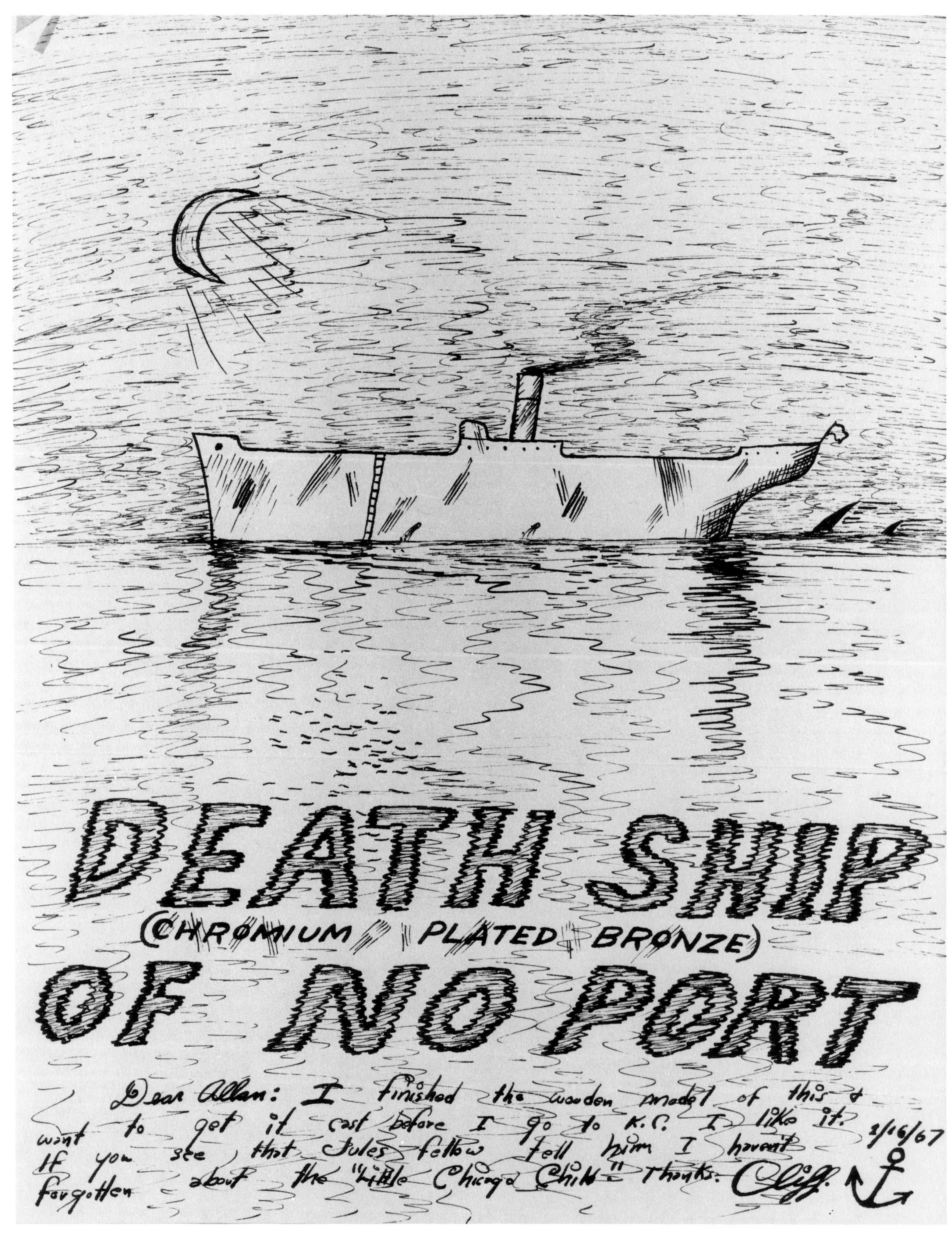
DEATH SHIP
(CHROMIUM PLATED BRONZE)
OF NO PORT
Dear Allan: I finished the wooden model of this &
want to get it cast before I go to K.C. I like it.
If you see that Jules fellow tell him I haven't
forgotten about the "Little Chicago Chill." Thanks. Cliff.
2/16/67

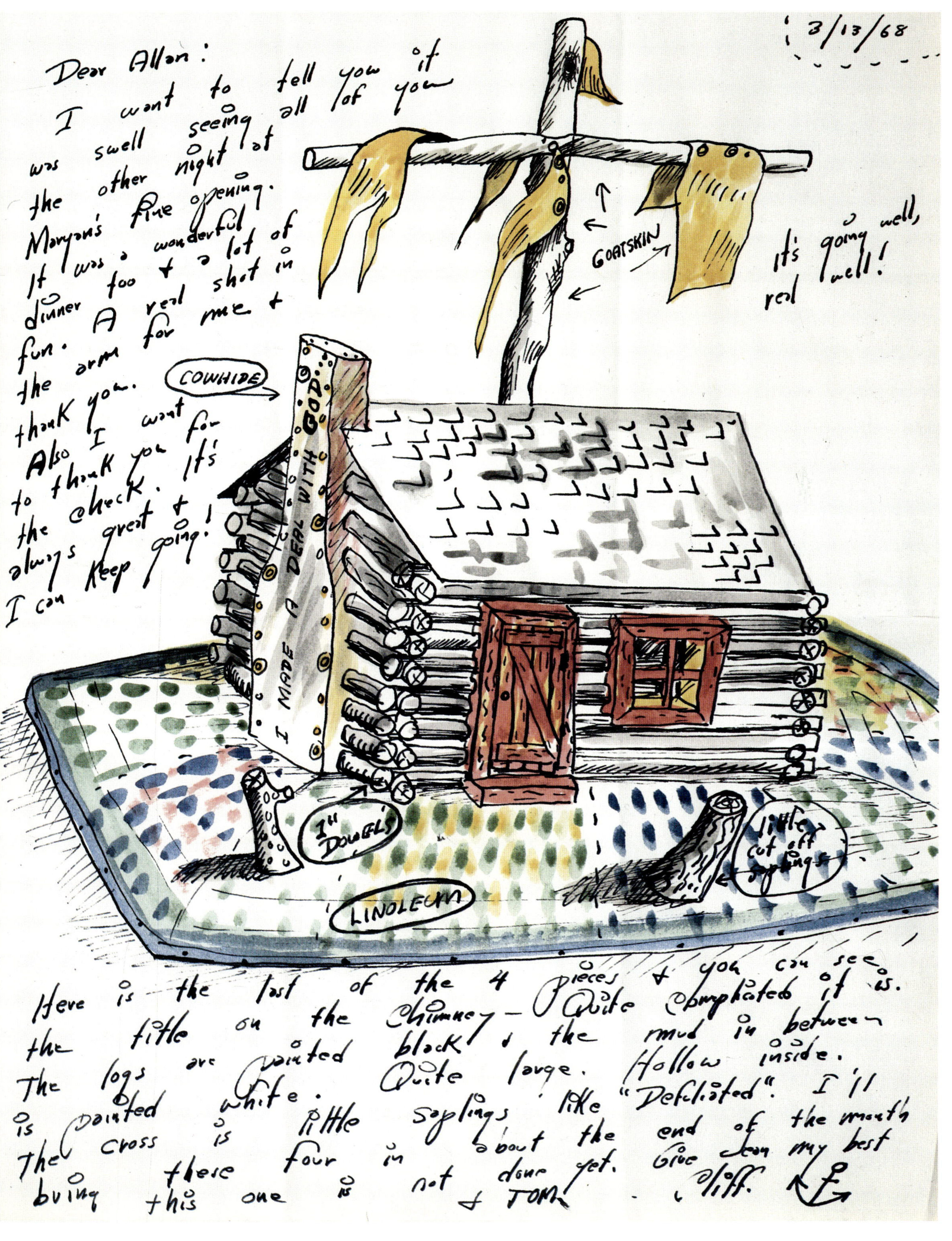

3/13/68

Dear Allan:

I want to tell you it was swell seeing all of you the other night at Maryon's fine opening. It was a wonderful dinner too + a lot of fun. A real shot in the arm for me + thank you. Also I want to thank you for the check. It's always great + I can keep going!

It's going well, real well!

Here is the last of the 4 pieces + you can see. Quite complicated it is. The title on the chimney + the mud in between the logs are painted black. Quite large. Hollow inside. The cross is painted white. little saplings like "Defoliated". I'll bring these four in about the end of the month + this one is not done yet. Give Jean my best + Tom.

Cliff.

October 20, 1969

Dear Allan:

I received the check + the bureaucracy that you signed + want to thank you for both. I've been thinking about you Allan + I just want to give you this piece. I made a piece earlier this year (well a box) for ole "rotten Rolf." I made a box present for Kenny Price too + one for Wiley. Well I've wanted to make you something + this piece (ill-fated spacecraft) is the one. I won't be offended in the least if you sell it + if you do, as it is a present don't figure it in the annual accounting, it's outside that + has nothing to do with the money you see. I just wanted to give you this to do with as you see fit. When I think about it you're the only one who has ever given me any dough + that means a lot to me. Well I hope you like this present, it came from where I live (the heart) ole friend + thanks for everything Allan. I'm going to sign my signature here so there won't be any question about this piece + its status in the future.

Cliff

November 4, 1976

Dear Allan:

I got your letter + the check + thank you. I'm sure glad the pieces arrived in Chi. in good order. Allan I hope you include all of the work, that I brought in, in the show there. I would appreciate that you hang all of the six watercolors that I brought in earlier in the year + of course all the woodcuts too. I'd appreciate it, after you hang the show to write + tell me exactly what is showing, you know a good description of it. It's hard for you to imagine but now all of that work that I brought in is gone now + I'll never see it again. It's a pretty shitty feeling. It's almost like it was flushed right down the toilet. You see, you don't have any idea what went into all of that. So please be careful with it anyway.

I've been thinking, all these years of the work I've done (+ it is on a level that absolutely nobody is aware of yet + probably never will be) except two people I know of. Anyway, the point being — I have very little to show for it, in the form of something really 1st class to look at myself + study. I think it would be a swell idea (+ it would help both of us) if at this stage you did a really first class catalogue. You know, very accurately + in depth + well written + mainly in color + you know color with my pieces + watercolors is very important. The only catalogue I have, in any depth at all, of course is the one from L.A. County Museum. That's not much to show for twenty years of very serious dedicated work. You mentioned possible shows with Jim later next year, Well that's OK with me. But I would like them <u>after</u> your show in the spring in N.Y., as you had planned.

I have been working on a new piece — no it's not the companion to the one-armed man. It's called "Fools Gold." In fact a couple of new ones. Allan when you get to Chicago would you kindly send my pal Dennis an announcement to my show. Of course I do intend to make some more boxes for the woodcuts + I will bring in some more sets of them.

Cliff

People in systems do not do what the system says they are doing.

Dec 28, 1976

Dear Richard:

That was a great surprise — that marvelous pork tenderloin. & Joanny & I cracked it open & started to work on it right away. It doesn't seem quite the same around here — or quite as nice, somehow, since you have moved away. Funny, because we never came up there to see you but once. We had a swell time though — Richard would you thank Jean for that lovely Christmas card she sent. I'm glad you got a good place to work in there & that K.C. is compatible with you & you can get the materials that you need to work with. Joanny & I are OK & we keep going. I had a big show in Chicago Nov 10 – Dec & have been working really good here since I finished my studio. Seven years to build that studio & outfit it — its a swell place

(2)

& it's the first place I've had to work in that was a good space & where I can have some order finally. That sure helps. I have a wood-burning stove in there & that works out perfect for heat. We have a lot of wood on our land here & I'm a pretty good wood-cutter. In fact I've got it down now to where it's an efficient operation & I don't do any fucking around. Richard I hope you & Jean had a swell Christmas & here's a toast to a grand New Year to the both of you!

Cliff

P.S. I really like that OCHS stamp!

The New York Times/Alan Riding

Peasants preparing to occupy land on a farm near Ciudad Obregón, Mexico

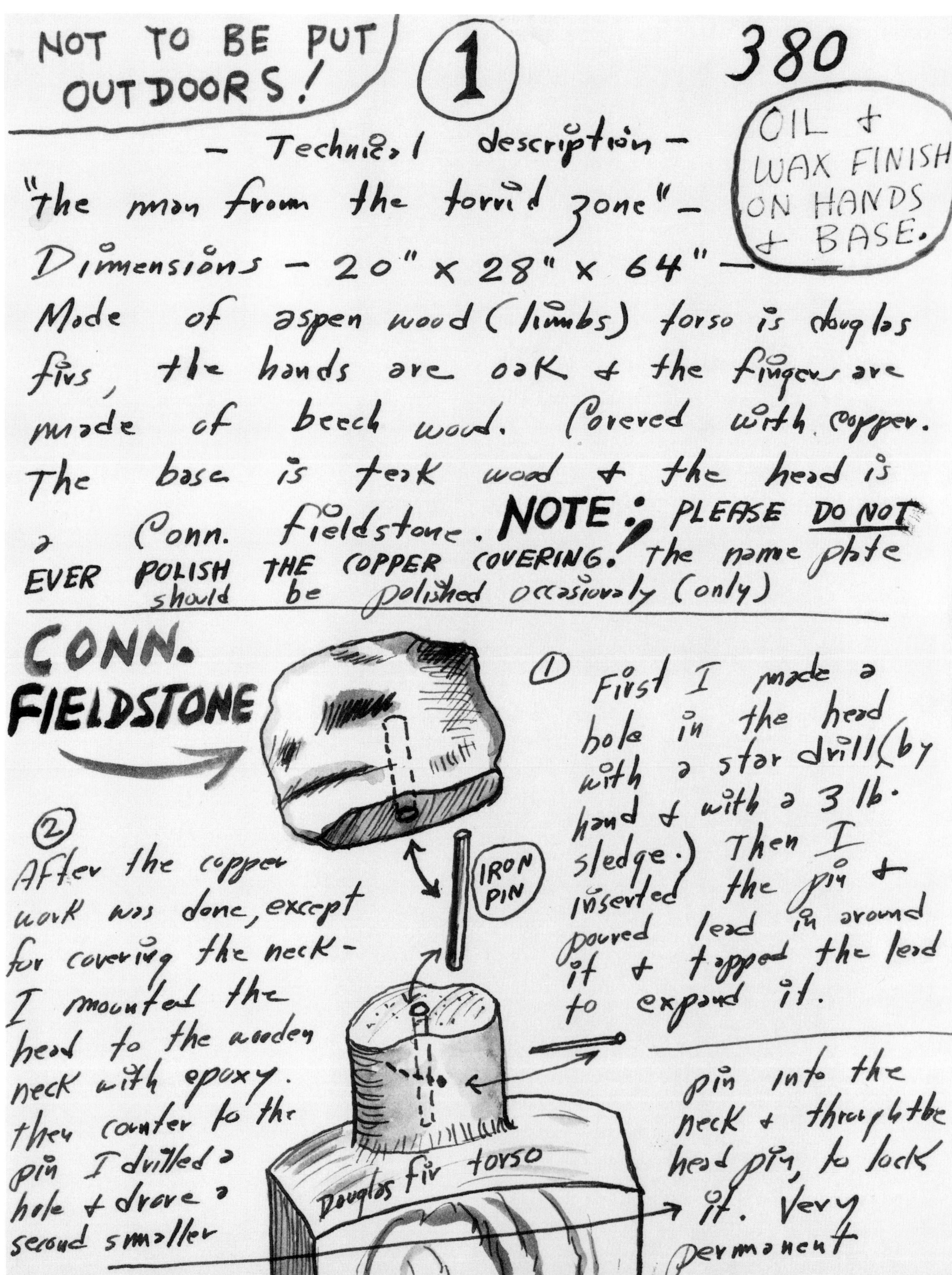

NOT TO BE PUT OUTDOORS!

1

380

OIL & WAX FINISH ON HANDS & BASE.

– Technical description –

"the man from the torrid zone" –

Dimensions – 20" x 28" x 64" –

Made of aspen wood (limbs) torso is douglas firs, the hands are oak & the fingers are made of beech wood. Covered with copper. The base is teak wood & the head is a Conn. fieldstone. **NOTE:** PLEASE DO NOT EVER POLISH THE COPPER COVERING! the name plate should be polished occasionally (only)

CONN. FIELDSTONE

① First I made a hole in the head with a star drill (by hand & with a 3 lb. sledge.) Then I inserted the pin & poured lead in around it & tapped the lead to expand it.

IRON PIN

② After the copper work was done, except for covering the neck – I mounted the head to the wooden neck with epoxy. then counter to the pin I drilled a hole & drove a second smaller pin into the neck & through the head pin, to lock it. Very permanent

Douglas fir torso

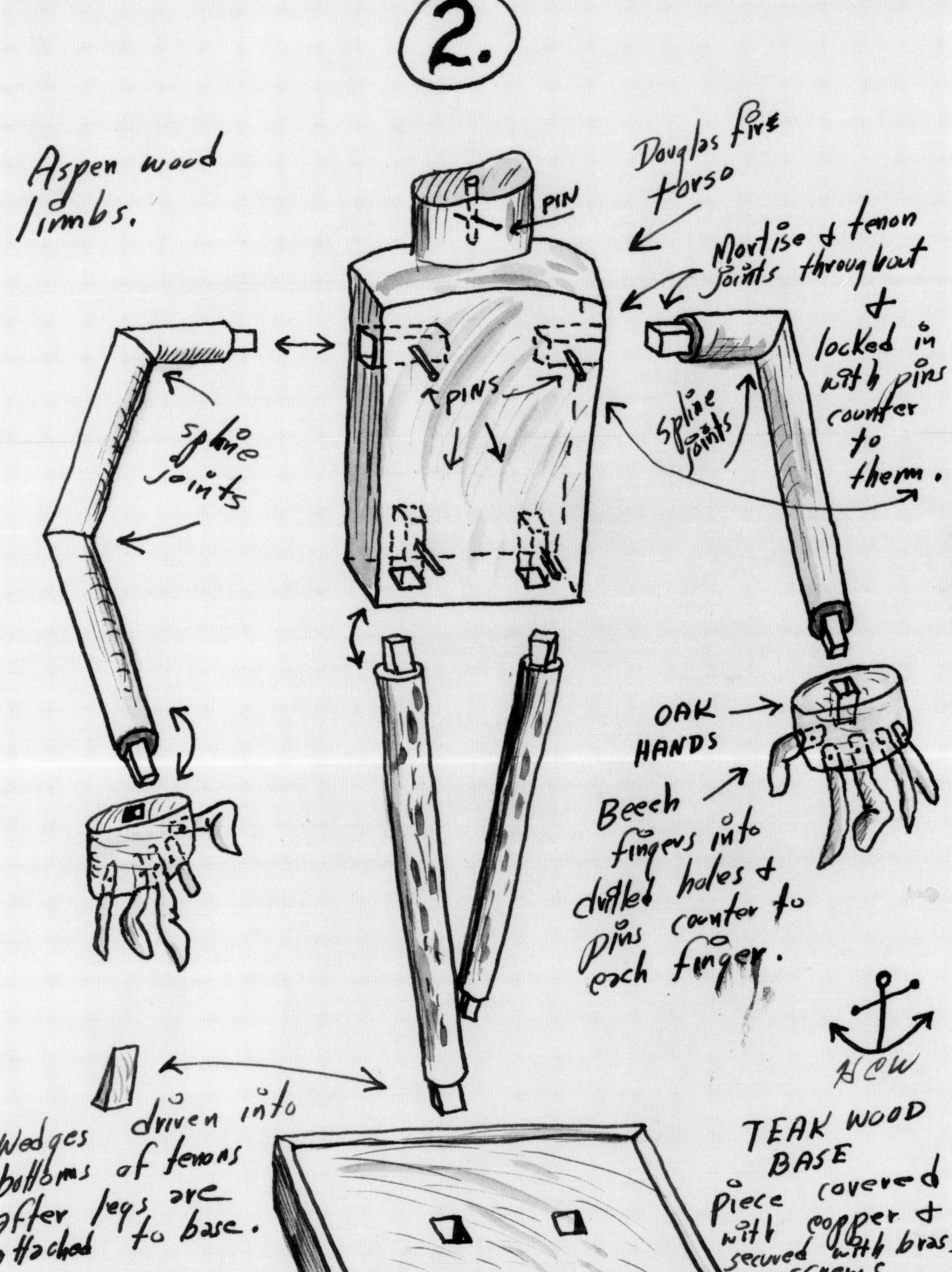
2.
Aspen wood limbs.
Douglas fire torso
PIN
Mortise & tenon joints throughout & locked in with pins counter to them.
PINS
spline joints
spline joints
OAK HANDS
Beech fingers into drilled holes & pins counter to each finger.
HCW
Wedges driven into bottoms of tenons after legs are attached to base.
TEAK WOOD BASE
Piece covered with copper & secured with brass screws

Joanna

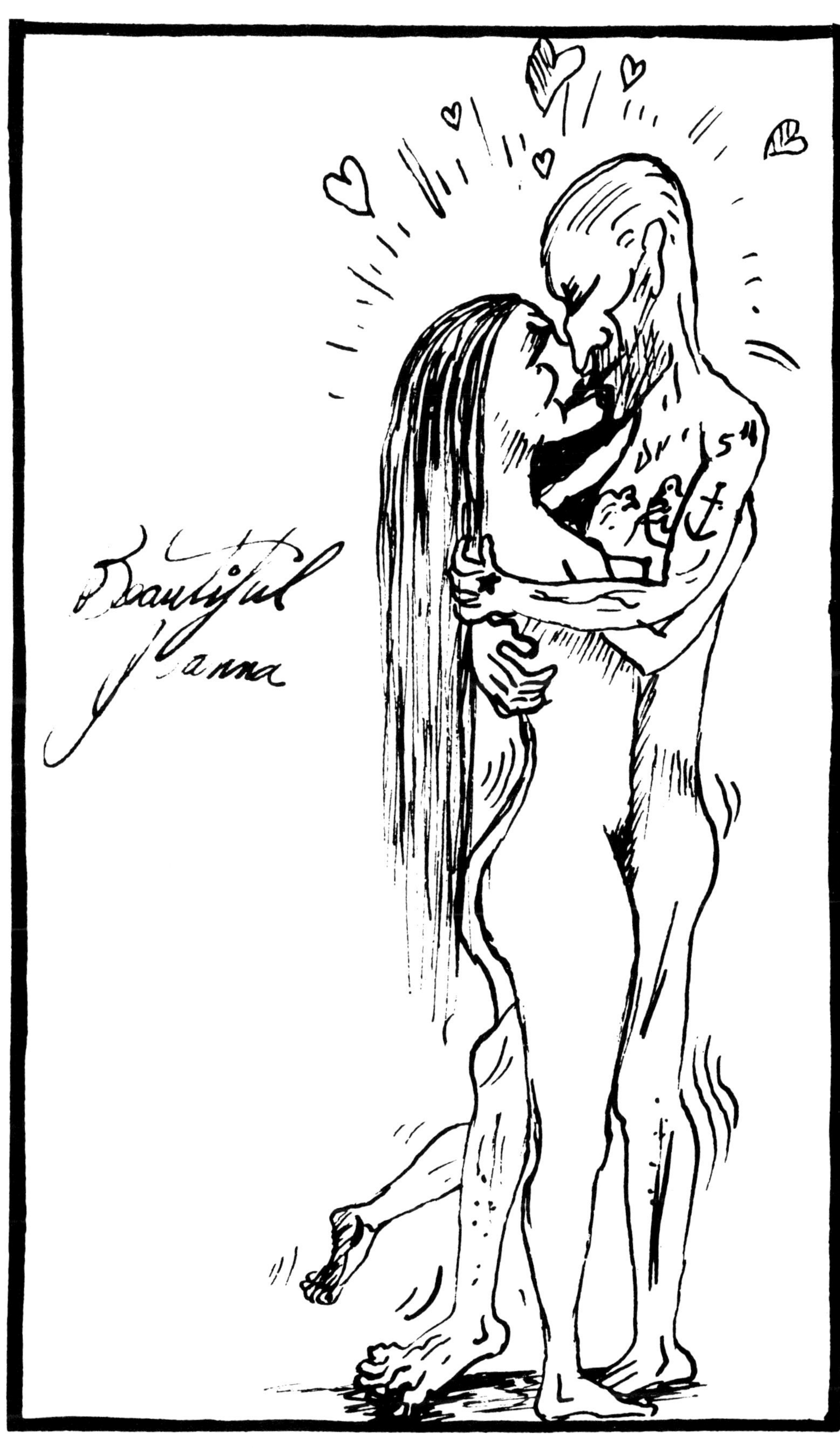

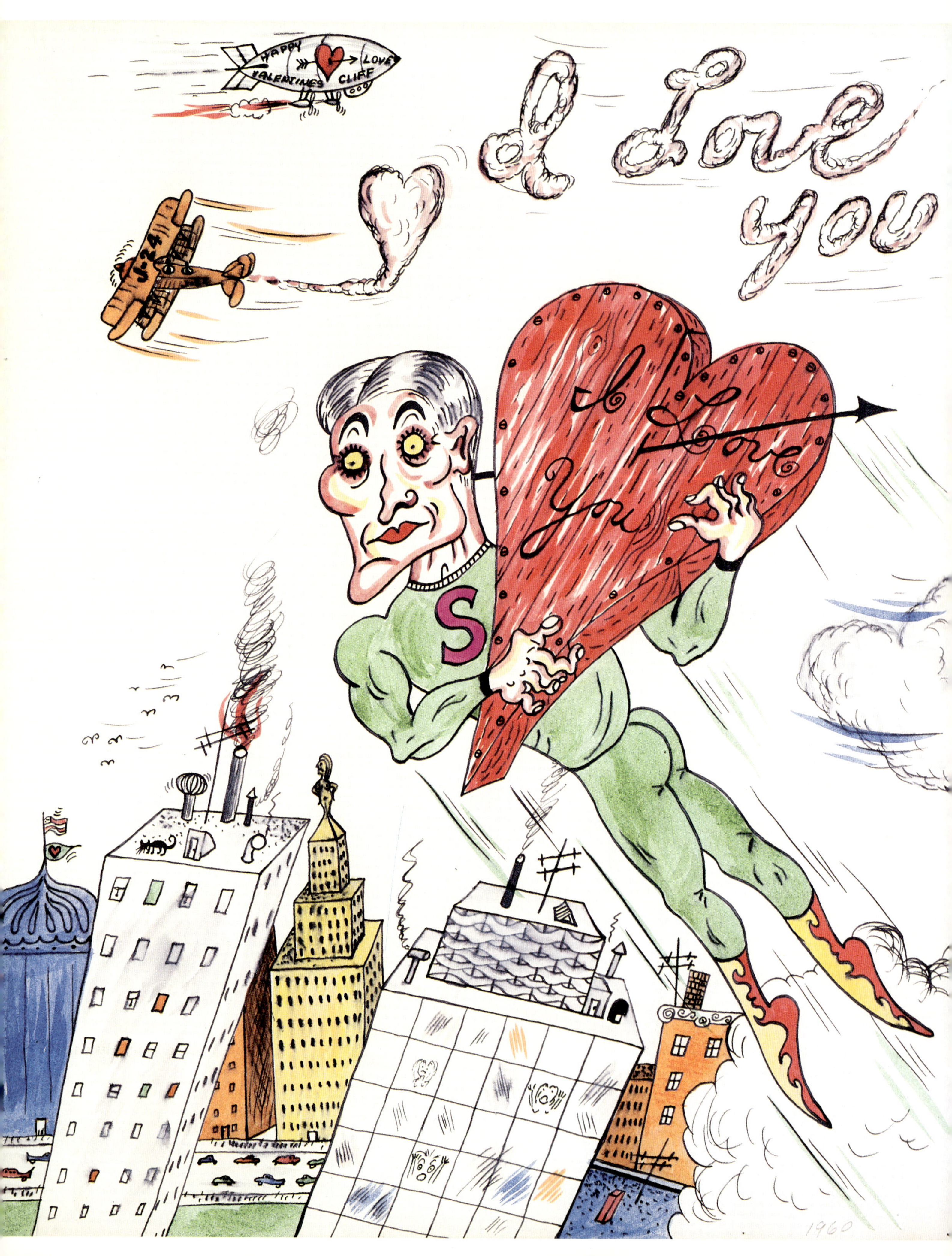
HAPPY VALENTINES
LOVE CLIFF
I Love you
J-24
I Love You
S
1960

Tues
May 16, '61

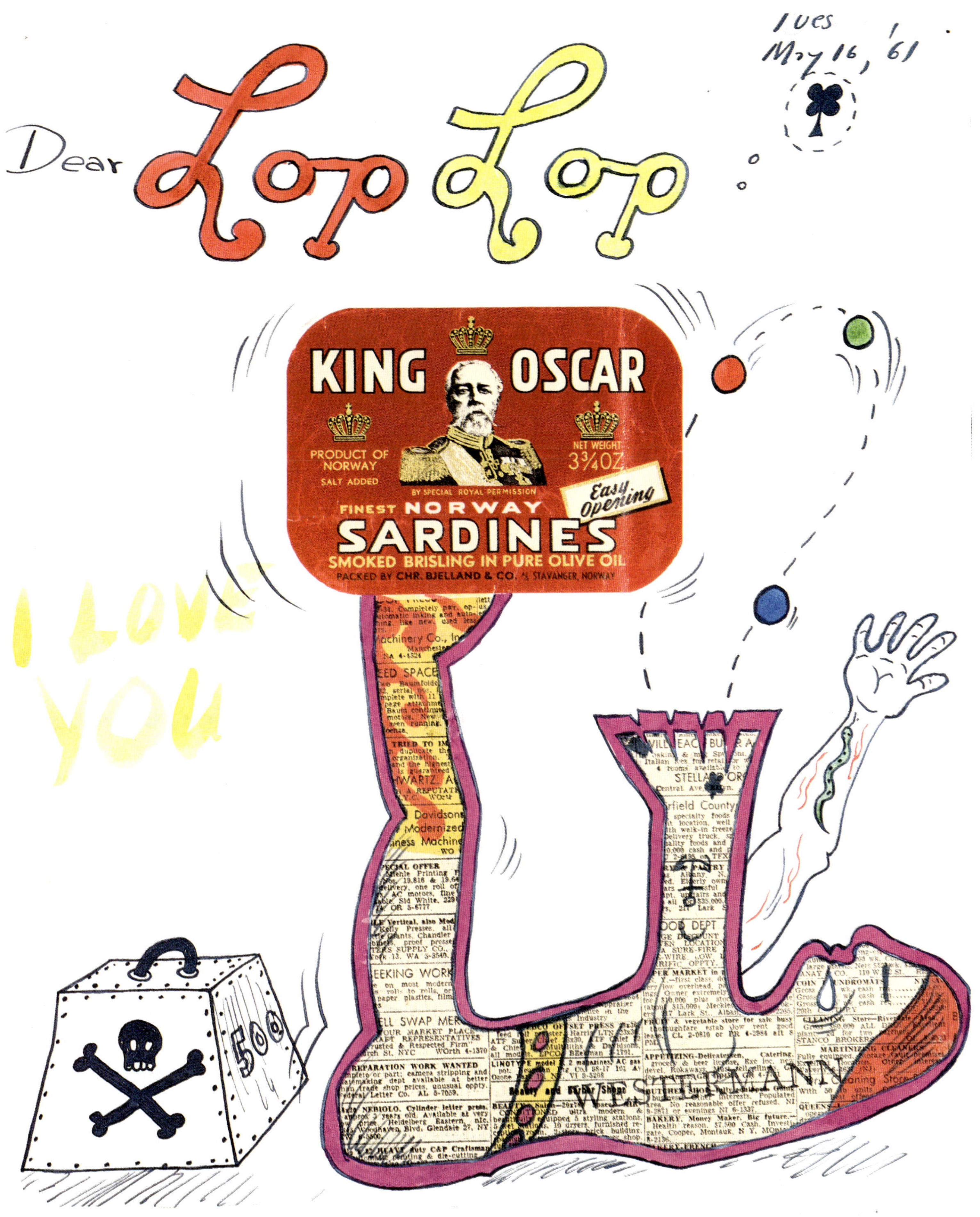

Tues.

Dear Mrs "Sweeda beed A":

It sure was good to talk to you tonight - Thanks for phoning you sure sounded great. I'll betcha yer glad to get away from my horrible "bitching" all the time! When we get back I'll promise to do better - I promise - That yellin is awful. I'm glad your eating. Now that the ole kitties are gone I'll finish up that can of "Puss-n-boots" & the "Cat yummies" HA HA. Sure miss you honey And miss looking across the table here at you like I'm doing now. No I've been eating - I threw a steak in the skillet with some eggs tonight & it was pretty good & I got a can of pineapple chunks too. I had a little left over so I cut them up & put them out on the back porch for ole Peco – he comes up here to see me once & a while. He's a nice ole guy & I think he misses his pals too. When I come back we'll go into N.Y. & see some movies & have a lot of fun & we'll go for walks around there. First I want to try and wind up the piece – Maybe Allan will get lucky h.h. Ole laughing boy

NOW CLIFFORD YOU DONT WANT TO GO TO CALIF.

100 $ 100

DEED

E.J.T. KEEP OUT

500 $ 500

OH MY GOD MY HEART – HELP HELP!

You know who this is ha, ha.

LOVE ♥ Always
CLIFF (MR SWAMI)

from a letter to Dorothy and Lester Beall June 10, 1959

However I could never forget to tell you Joanna is a wonderful wonderful, gentle, fine little woman, and she's all woman too. No man ever had a finer wife than she's been and I've a real need for her. She helps me in every way and she's certainly given life a fuller + finer meaning. I wish you could see her as my wife and you would see this also. She has a great spirit + determination + she's very courageous. And boy oh boy can she cook beautifully. Well I'm very, very, happy with her + know a happiness I didn't believe was possible before.

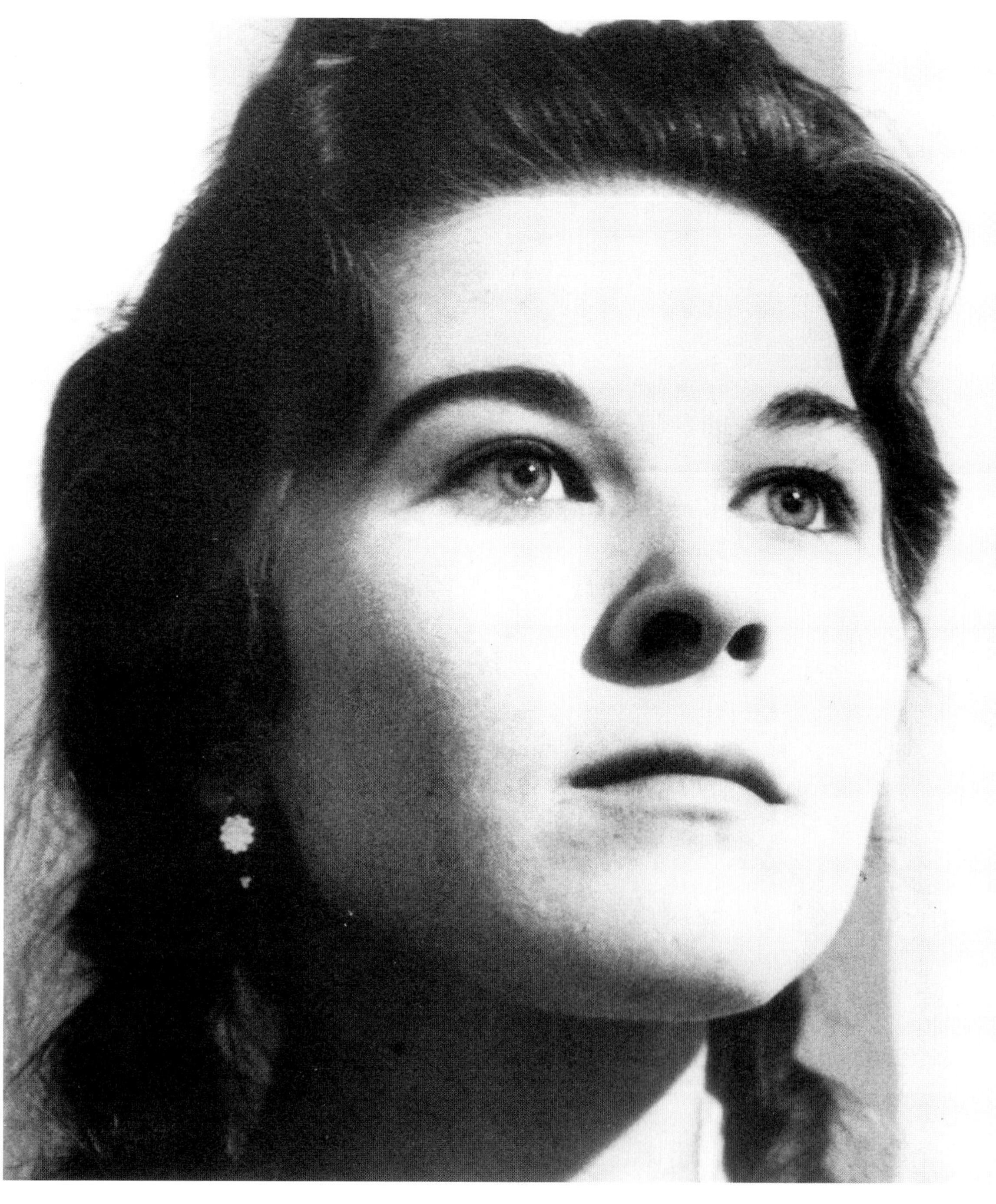

Joanna Beall Westermann photographed by Westermann, 1962

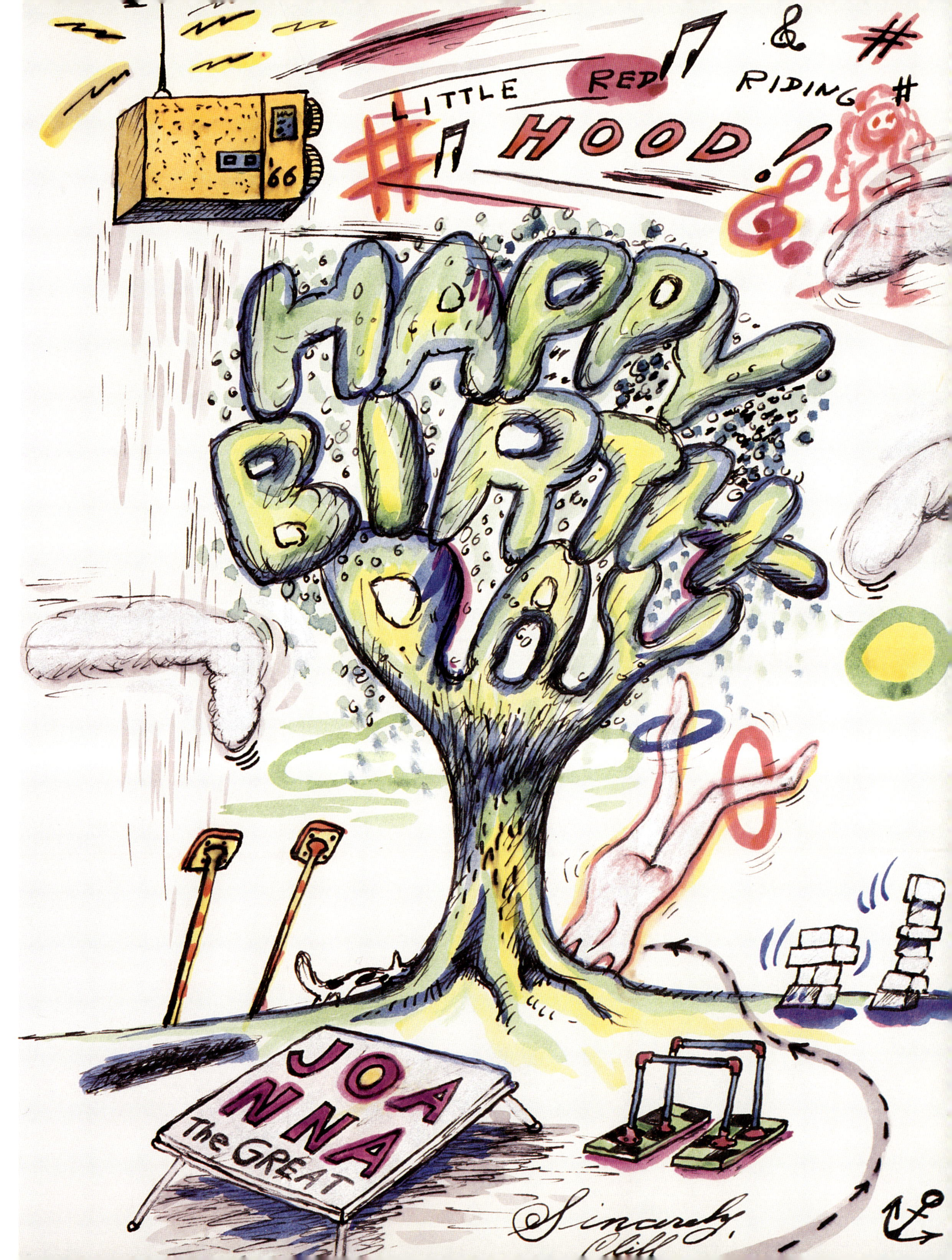

'66
LITTLE RED RIDING
HOOD!
HAPPY BIRTHDAY
JOANNA
The GREAT
Sincerely,

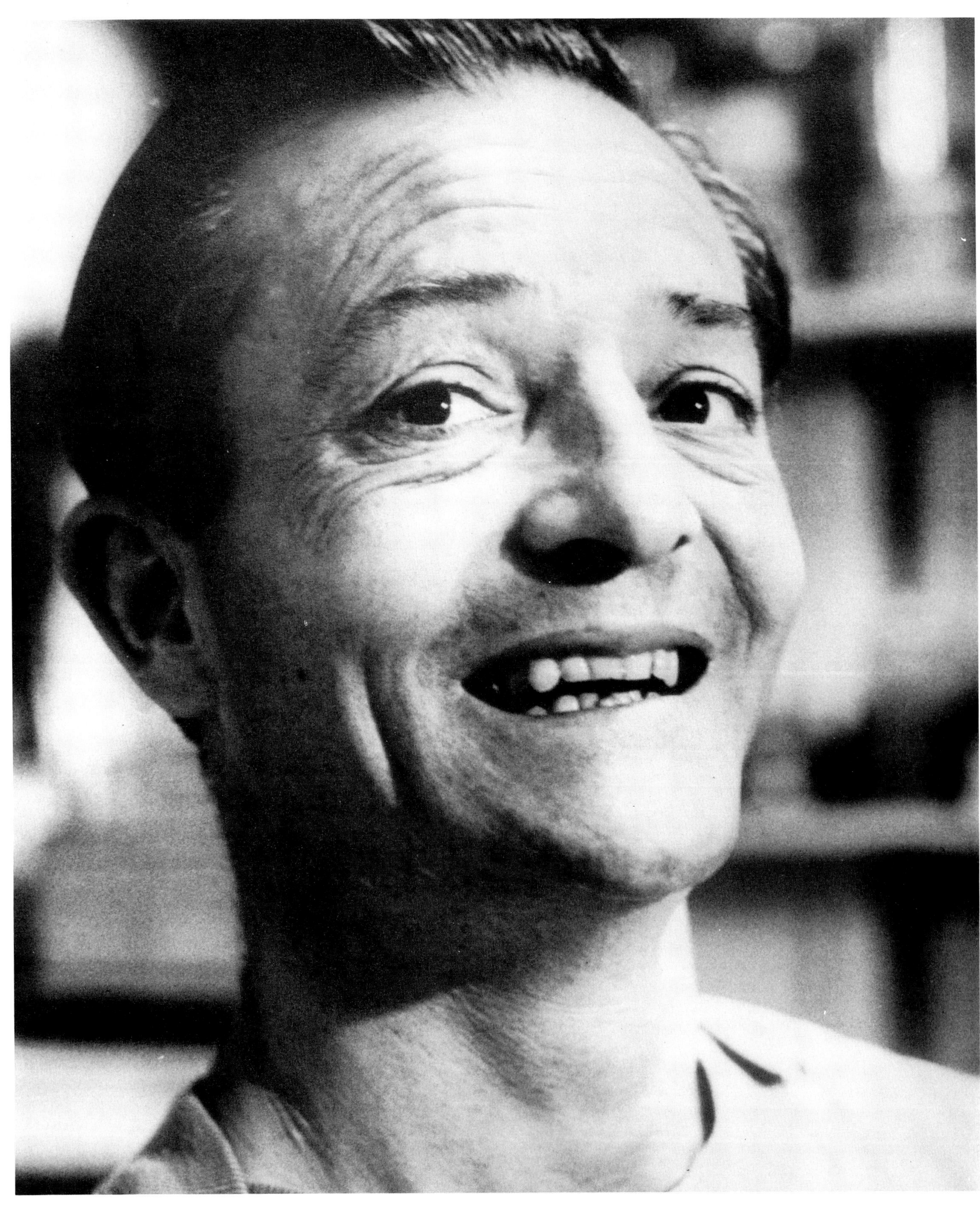

Westermann photographed by Joanna Beall Westermann, 1962

HI YA SWEETHEART!!

Joanna Dear

FRI

all

My Beloved little Balancer:
Aren't I a silly shit with
my dumb little drawings & boring
you to death with all these
letters? I'm sorry —

please darling, use
any of the money for
nice things for yourself,
clothes, art gear,
pty rocks,
etc.

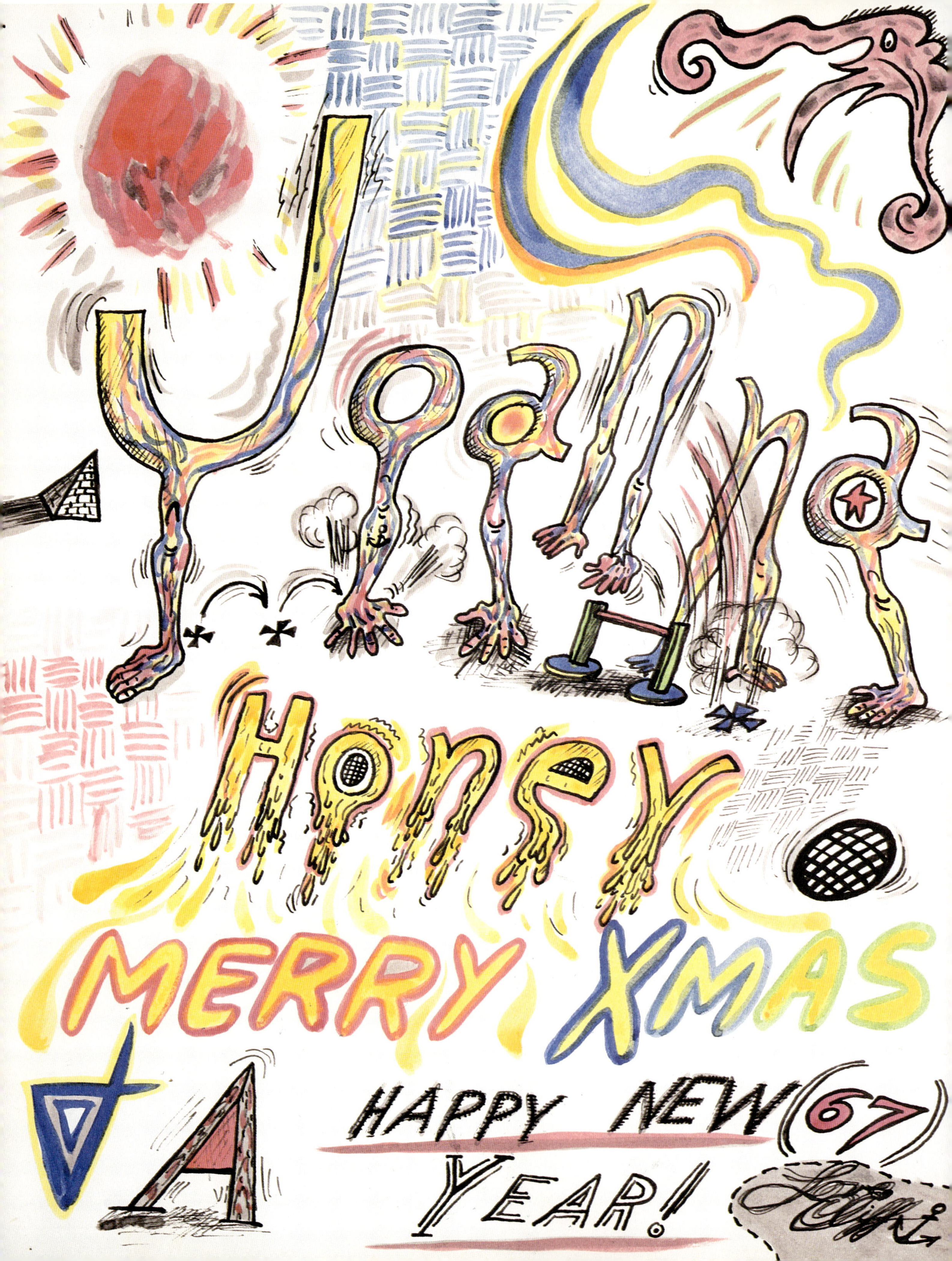

Honey
MERRY XMAS
HAPPY NEW (67) YEAR!

Thursday (1968)

Dear Love will find a way:

I got your wonderful letter. I love them! You gotta keep your eye on needle dink the bug f---------!!! And I'm so glad "General" is coming home next Tues. Gee I'll bet he'll be glad. Yesterday morning as I started to Tamarind there I saw a fat wallet out in the middle of the street. I mean fat, like there was 10,000 $ in it. So I dove for it and it contained 4 $ and about 15 snapshots of girlfriends in color. All inscribed "To Lin with love" — "Love forever", etc. It seems ole Lin is a student at UCLA and you could plainly see what he was majoring in. His full name was Lin Carter Tang (I called him "poon-tang" for short) And he lived right near here. Also was a girlie address book with more broads' addresses about 100 of them. + drivers license, credit cards, etc. After Tamarind last night I took the wallet over to the young man's house and gave it to his brother as he was not at home. Funny!! He was probably out with a girlfriend. I guess Tamarind will shape up — it was better. I sure love you and miss you sweet heart.

Love,
Your Little Husband

Sunday October 20, 1968

My Dearest Beloved Little Wife + Pal:

If I were in a big room with 10,000 women + you were amongst them + I had not met you before + then suddenly saw you for the first time in my life — Why I would just walk over to my baby, kiss you, take your little hand in mine + just walk away from all those broads with you — my true sweetheart! + that is the truth. + we would just go away by ourselves + live happily ever after in the woods with kitties + racks + a dog maybe + all the crowsys + birds. Wouldn't that be something. Just baby + me!

Yesterday (Sat.) Maurice Tuchman, Jim Monte, the catalog designer, + some other people from the museum came up to the apt to discuss the show etc. It looked to me like they were all trying to get out of something dis-tasteful to them. They asked to see some drawings I had made for the lithos + they didn't say a fuckin' word about them. Even if they had said they were shit, it would have been something. Museum people are all busier than hell doing nothing + very bored too. I don't like them. They were all going someplace, flying, Monday morning, a big nothing. Big deals + big nothing + boy how they hate the artists. Hey sweetheart I learned, finally, how to do a walkover. It just came natural + I even learned it up here in the apt, when I was taking a workout the other night. The living room up here is large enough to workout in. I've done hundreds of headstands since I been here. I hope you still kick a few every day honey. They really are good for you, I think. I'll always have a picture of you in my mind doing laps, jogging, around our little oval. "Cuter than a bug's ear"!!! I think Allan is pissed off about giving me a raise. Now he's going to have to go to work a little, ha, ha, ha. I LOVE YOU!!

Love,
"White Cloud"

I always
loved halloween
with baby!

November 18, 1968

Dearest Sweetheart:

Wow you are really uncanny, because every time I wish I had + really need a letter from you, like magic there's one in my ole #308 box — Wow!!! I don't know how you know but there it is. When I got back late last night from Martha's there it was — thanks honey. I sure love hearing from you — that's the next to the best thing of all, you sweet. It was good seeing Martha + Mike again + their kids + they all said to say hello to you. I didn't leave their house the whole weekend + got looking at old things. Martha gave me mother's old postcard album to look at + a little book that she wrote in all about their marriage in 1920. You know, gifts received, the marriage, the honeymoon, etc. + of course the "great expectations". Well the book really tore me apart + was the saddest thing I ever read plus the photo album too. It was terribly sad — it was too much! I'm glad you didn't read it. Carl Bloom was one best man at their wedding. They had a little reception at their house in Muskogee afterwards + nobody showed up + my poor mother said well it must have been because it was a "rainy day". How terrible. They both looked so sad in their wedding picture + in their snapshots before + after they were married + they were both so beautiful + young. Oh my God. Gee I'll sure be glad to get back to my baby + it won't be so long now. I love you.

Love,
Your Little Husband

November 22, 1968

My Beautiful Girl:

"Prettiest girl I ever did see"!! Yesterday Rolf came to the museum + brought the beautiful collage you had made for him. WOW!!!! Honey you're really sitting on it — Doing beautiful things! Gee I sure loved that + Rolf is so proud of it — He's going to get it framed immediately!!! Nobody can do those collages like you — really honey. I'm still working on the pieces at the museum + should finish them today. They weren't too bad, just filthy dirty + I think the museum would have gone ahead + shown them anyhow without even cleaning the glasses. I really think the whole thing with the show has been pretty shoddy + I'm quite disappointed with it honey. For one the exhibition room is too small etc. etc. + then the catalog is 3rd rate. What's odd about the whole thing though is the museum people think it's a swell job, including the catalog. I just don't think they know any better. There is about as much enthusiasm to work around here as there is in a factory (+ that's what it is, really). Very unprofessional. But you wouldn't be surprised honey. I think the museums + their attitudes are all alike now. Something like insurance people or bankers or used car dealers — SHIT - SHIT - SHIT - PEW. Anyway I hate that + it's not the way. But I sure love you honey + miss you all the time.

Love,
Big C

Allan is arriving
TODAY — up Tight

April '71

Dearest Sweety:

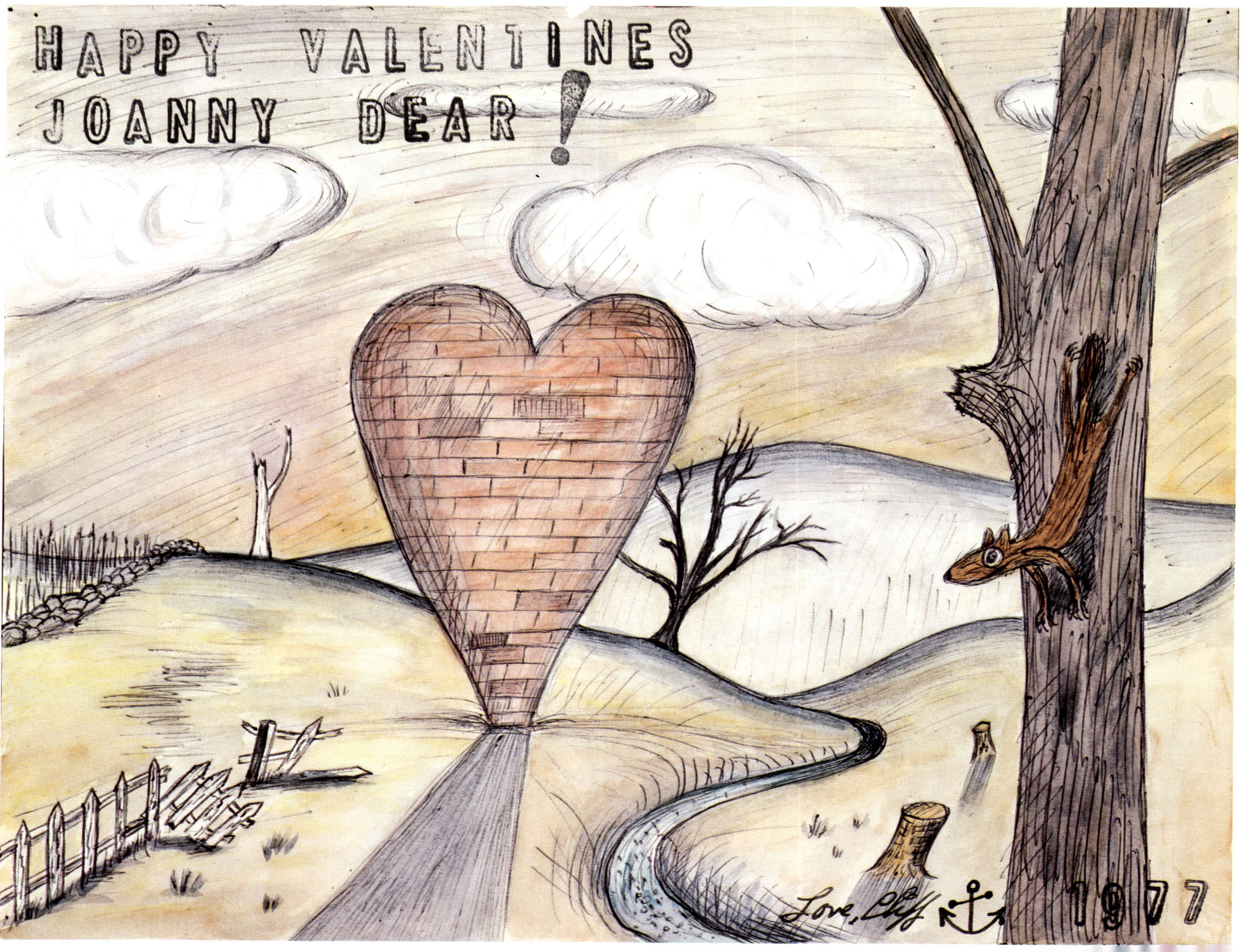
HAPPY VALENTINES
JOANNY DEAR!
Love, Cliff
1977

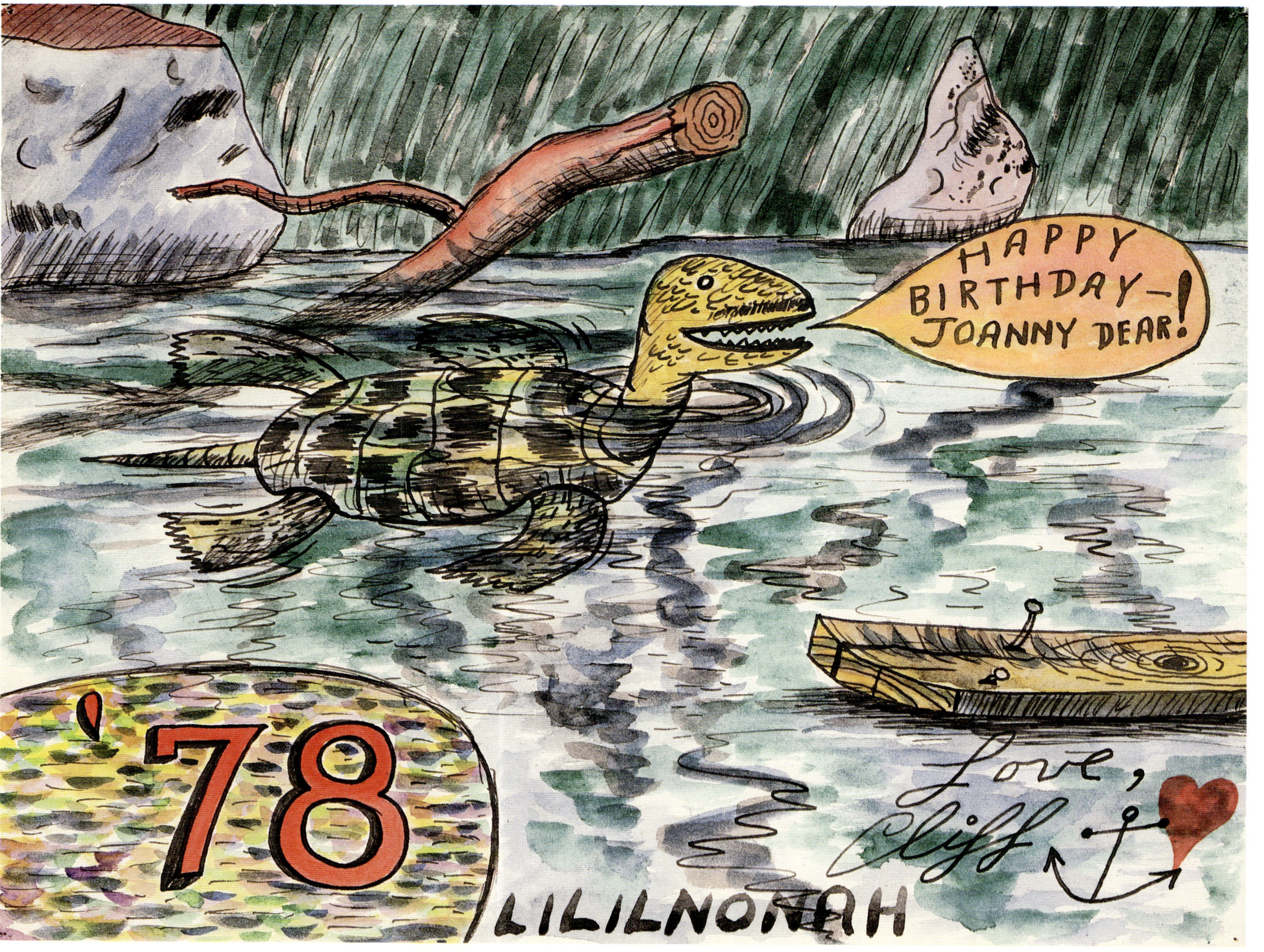
HAPPY BIRTHDAY— JOANNY DEAR!
'78
LILILNONAH
Love,
Cliff

A Country Gone Nuts

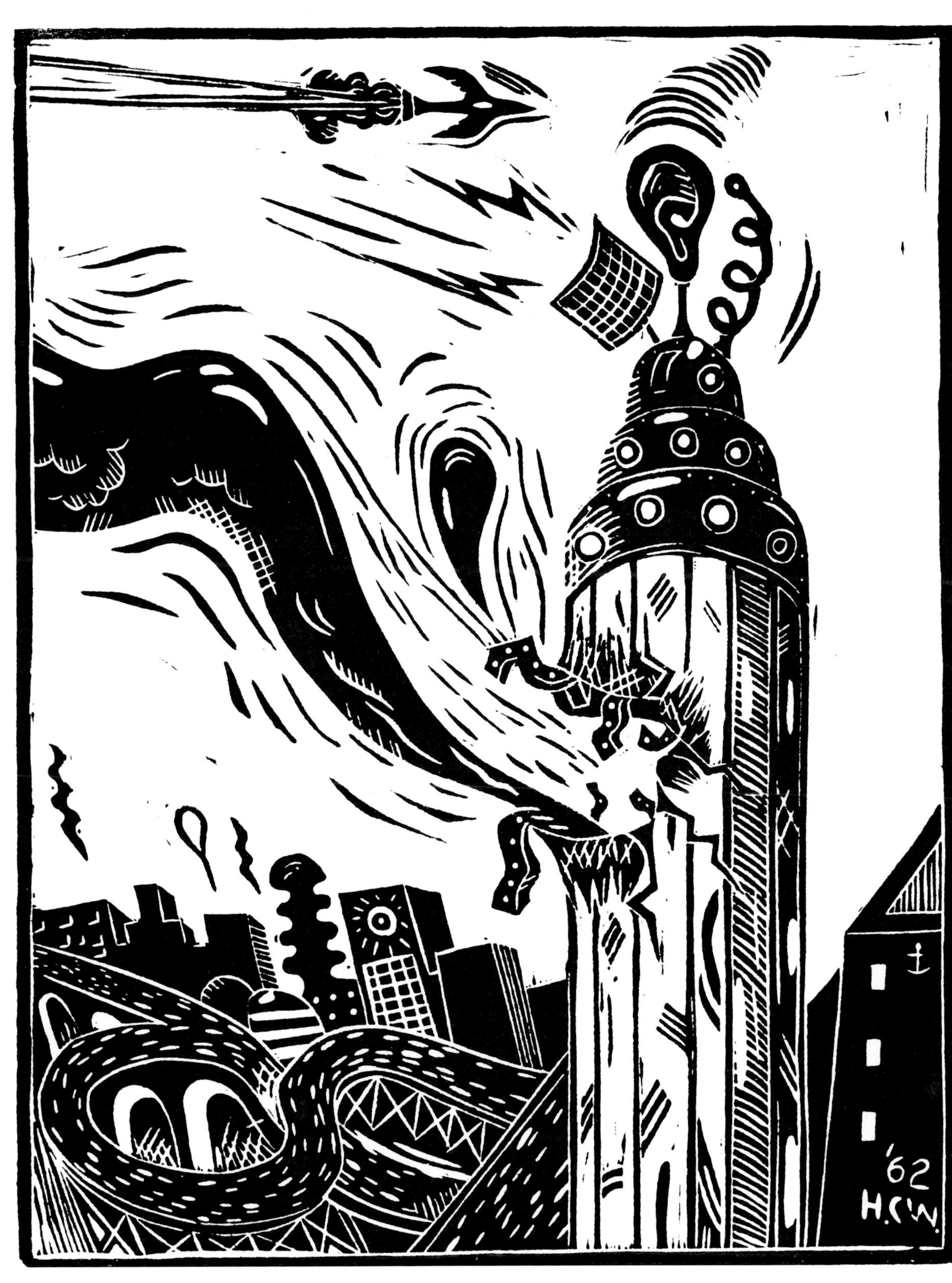

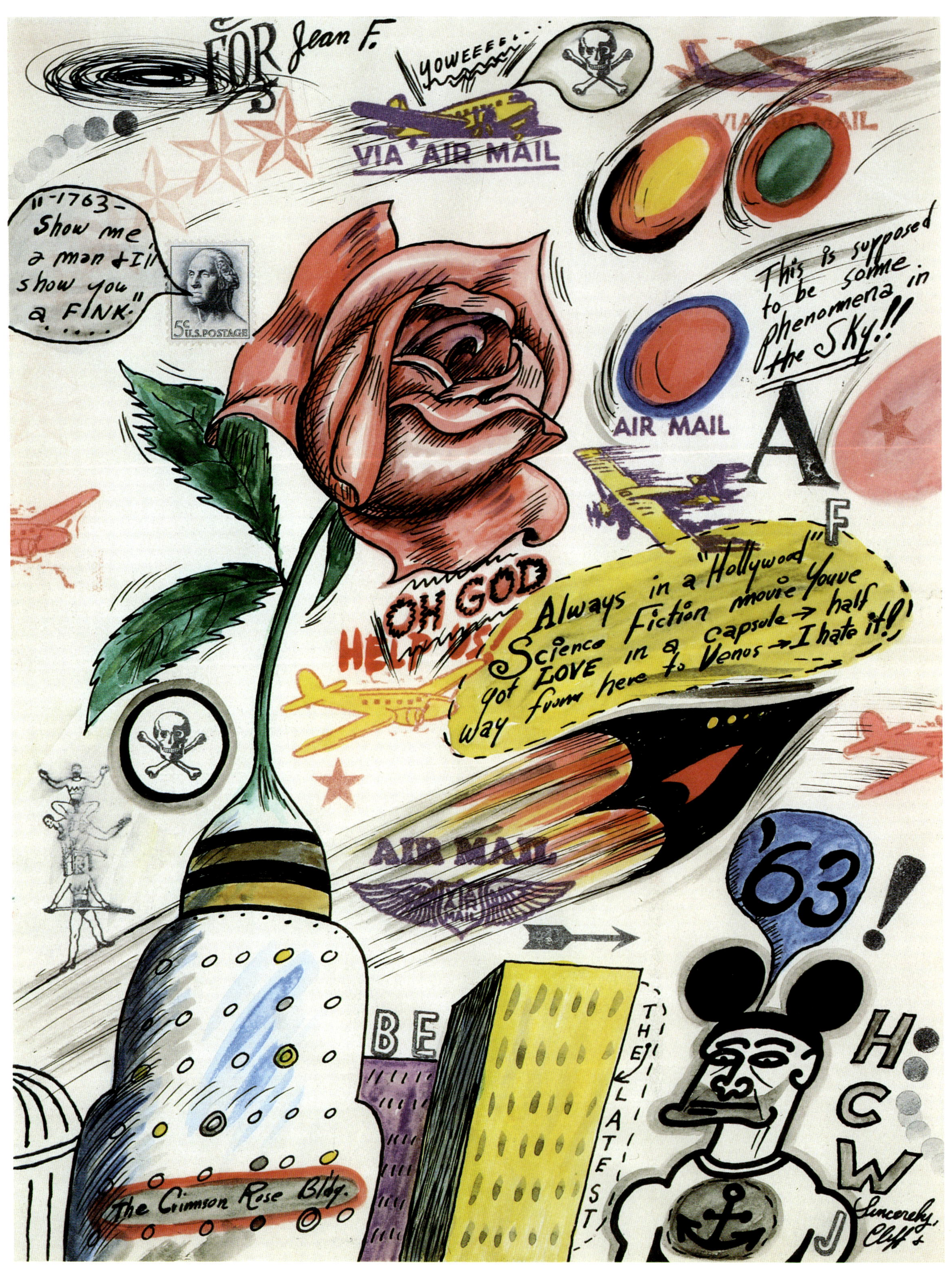FOR Jean F.
YOWEEEE.....
VIA AIR MAIL
11-1763- Show me a man + I'll show you a FINK"....
5¢ U.S. POSTAGE
This is supposed to be some phenomena in the Sky!!
AIR MAIL
A
F
OH GOD
HELP US!
Always in a "Hollywood" Science Fiction movie Youve got LOVE in a capsule → half way from here to Venos → I hate it!!
AIR MAIL
VIA AIR MAIL
'63!
BE
THE LATEST
H
C
W
J
The Cimson Rose Bldg.
Sincerely, Cliff +

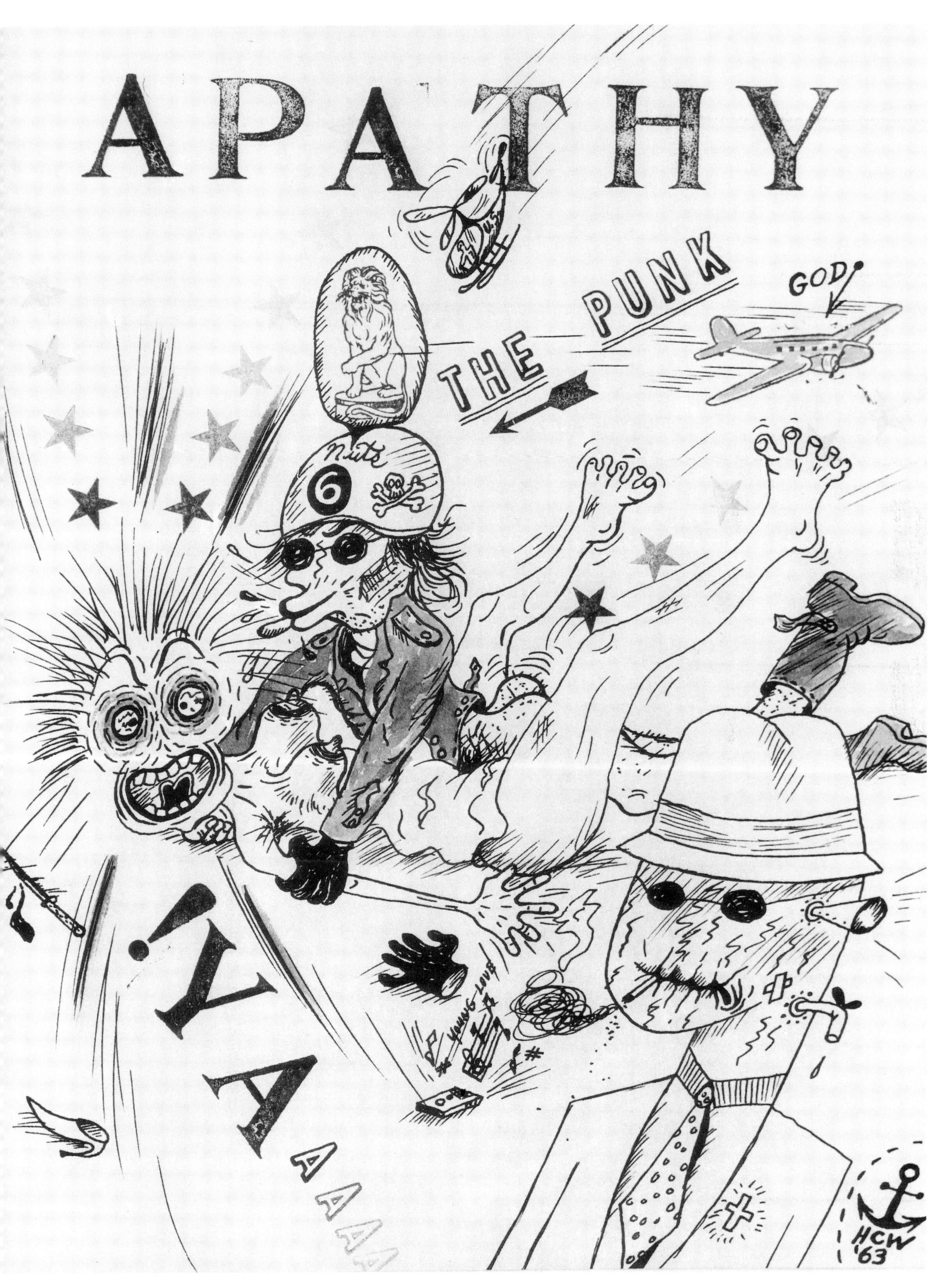
APATHY
THE PUNK
GOD
YOUNG LOVE
HCW '63

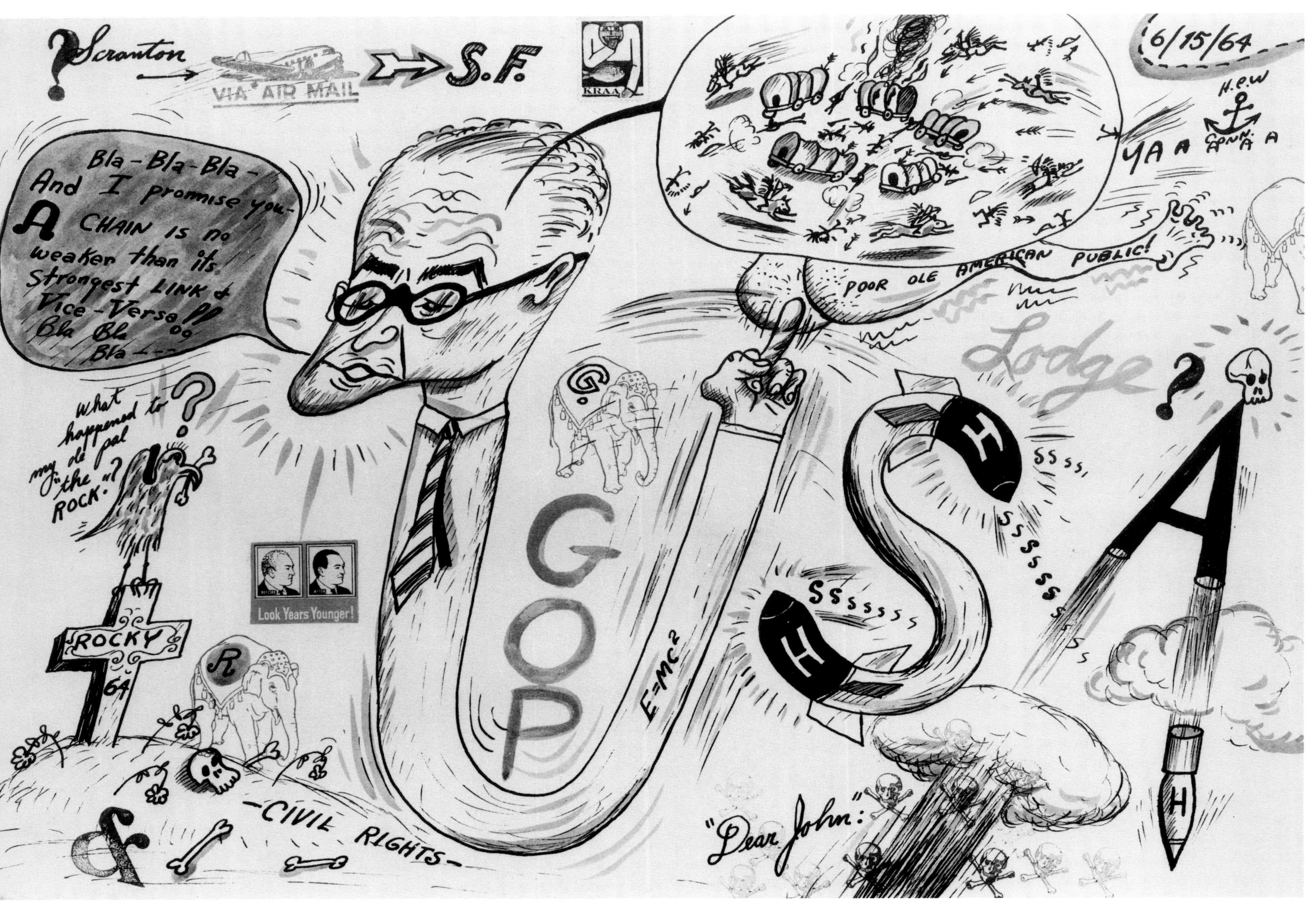
Scranton → VIA AIR MAIL → S.F.
KRAA
6/15/64
Bla-Bla-Bla-
And I promise you-
A CHAIN is no weaker than its Strongest LINK & Vice-Versa!!
Bla Bla Bla
What happened to my ole pal "the ROCK"?
ROCKY 64
Look Years Younger!
POOR OLE AMERICAN PUBLIC!
Lodge?
H.E.W
YAA
GOP
E=MC²
USA
-CIVIL RIGHTS-
"Dear John:"

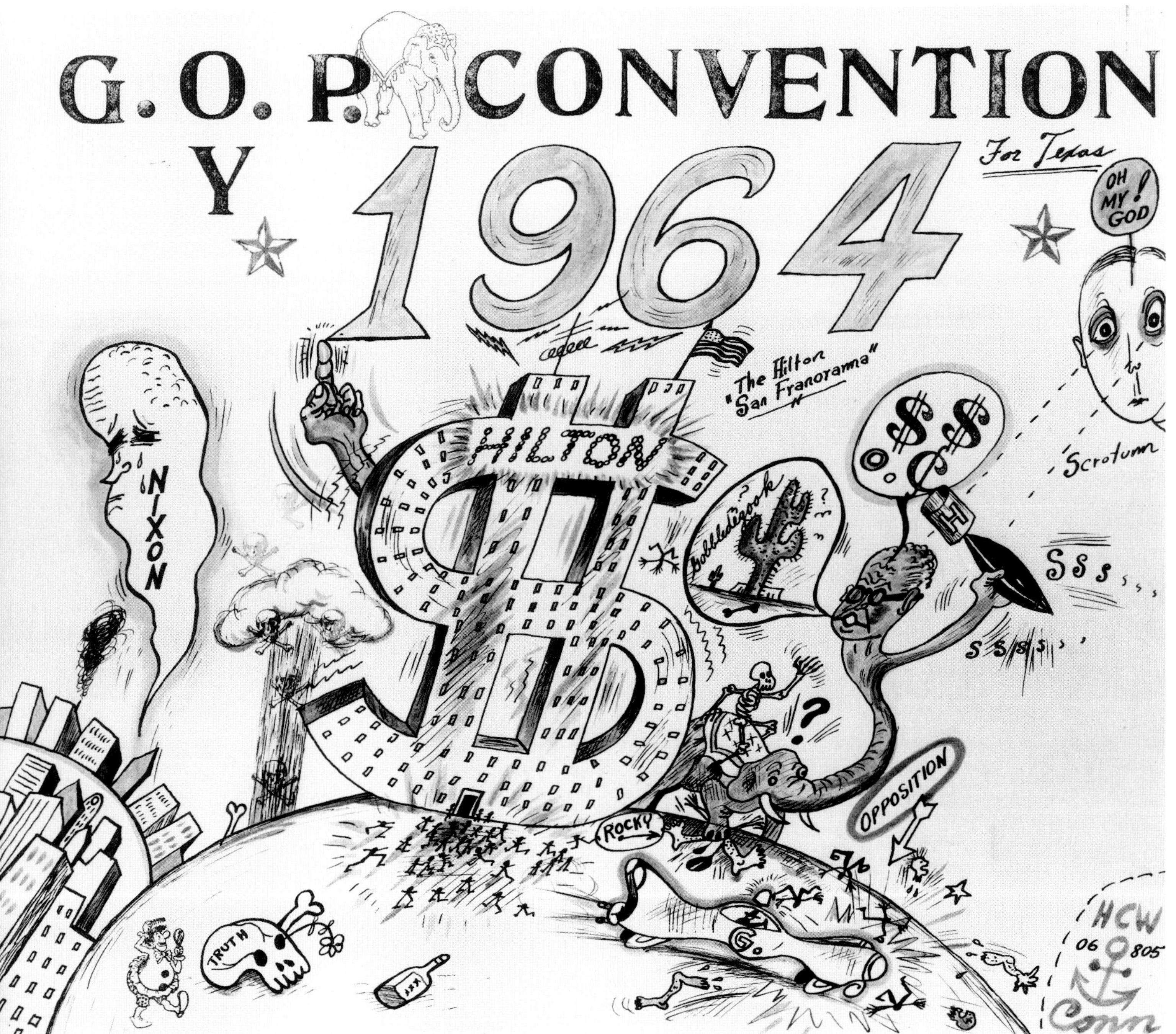

from a letter to Allan Frumkin June 29, 1964

Earlier this month I got a letter from Jim Newman asking me if I would draw a picture for his G.O.P. convention show. He said he'd like one. Well I got pretty excited with the theme + made four (4) of them + sent them to him. They turned out pretty raw so I doubt whether he can use them. I suppose he will send them on to you after the show.

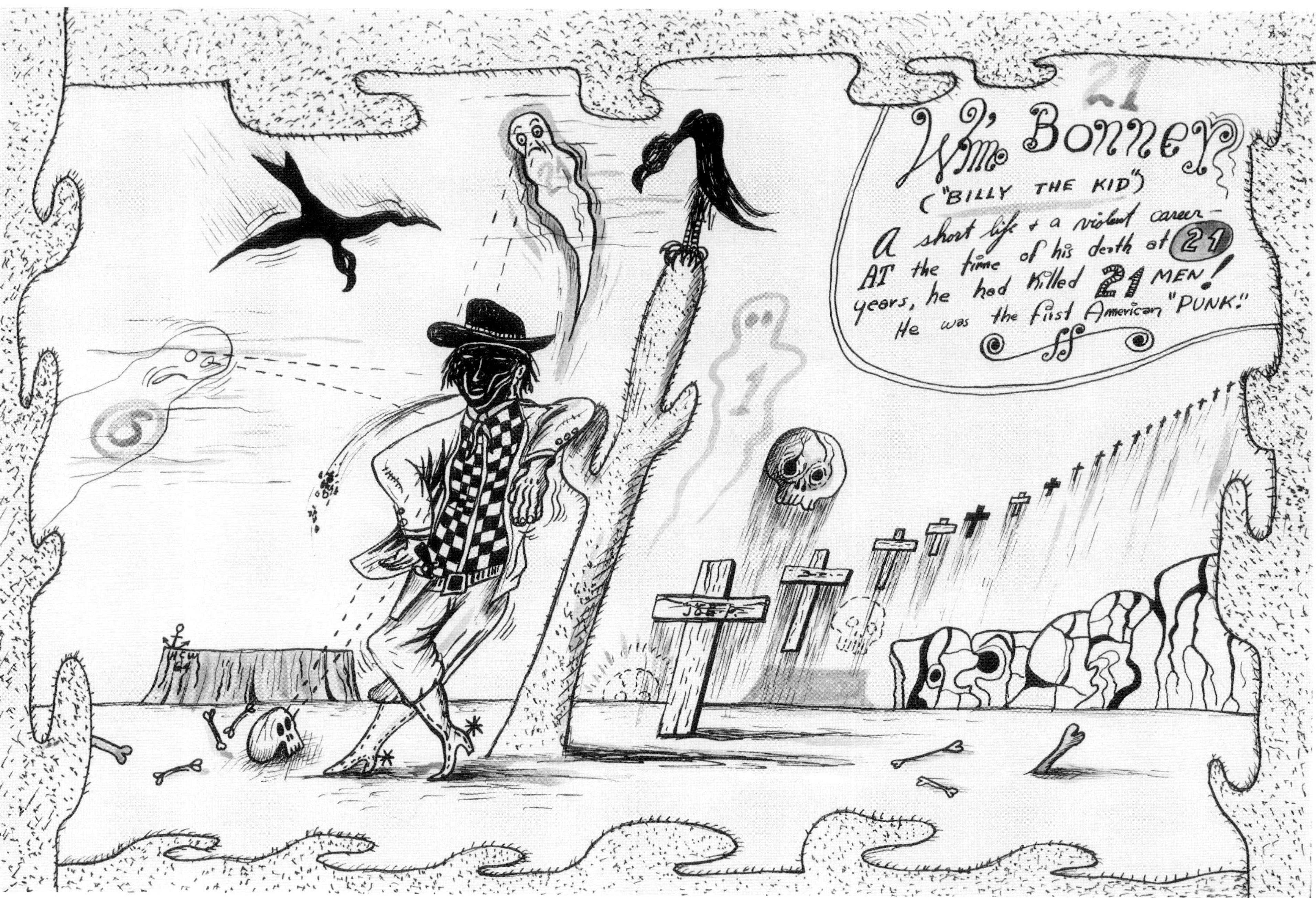
Wm. Bonney
("BILLY THE KID")
A short life & a violent career—
AT the time of his death at 21
years, he had killed 21 MEN!
He was the first American "PUNK!"
JOE P.

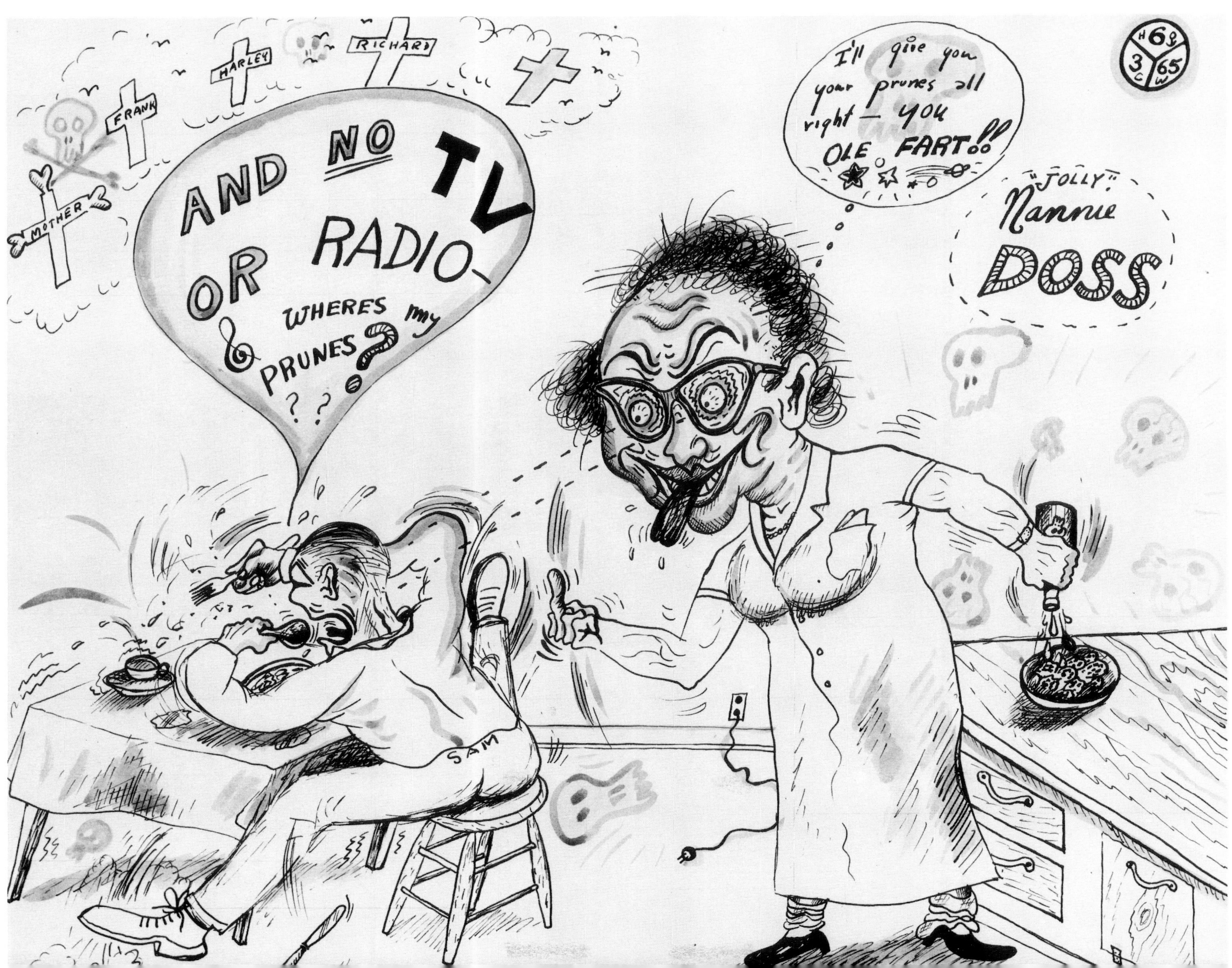
MOTHER
FRANK
HARLEY
RICHARD
AND NO TV OR RADIO — & WHERES my PRUNES???
SAM
I'll give you your prunes all right — YOU OLE FART!!
"JOLLY" Nannie DOSS
H 6 ♀ 3 C 65 W

Suicide Rehearsal, Death in 'Costume'

A 41-year-old ex-seaman who meticulously planned his "final curtain" to the point of compiling lists of items required and staging careful suicide rehearsals—was found dead here yesterday.

The victim, Raymond J. Denne, was found by his landlady in his shabby apartment at 1097 McAllister street—hanging from a noose attached to the wall by an eye hook, with his hands bound tightly behind him with rope in handcuff fashion. His legs were bound with a pair of suspenders and his mouth gagged with a pair of women's panties.

He was dressed in a black woman's evening gown, patent leather shoes, nylons and a brassiere.

NOTES

The final notes in his big ledger-type diary, which were made Thursday, about the time of his death, said:

"This is it. I've had it . . . Police Department, please see I am buried in clothing laid out on bed (standard men's clothing—slacks, shirt, shoes). I am not a queer. Just had a compulsion to wear this 'costume' to die in.

"Good-by, world. The next one can't likely be much worse."

Police Inspector Walter Kracke said a homicide investigation would continue "pending the outcome of handwriting analysis."

DOUBTS

Deputy Coroner Mark Alleeson said, "I don't see how it could be (a suicide). If it was, it's the most ingenious I've ever seen."

On the bed was a list of the suicide items he had used. One item on the list was "falsies," but that was crossed out, with the word "scrapped" beside it.

The diary was a long recounting of frustrations, said Inspector Kracke. Denne had quit his seaman's life about the first of the year—when he started the diary—and began looking for work on land. He worked briefly as a stockboy, then was fired or quit.

GIRLS

He wrote additionally of two girl friends who were transvestites and who apparently had affairs with women as well as with him.

References to the "final curtain" began appearing about February.

The entry for March 29 read: "Stayed and rehearsed a bit more without dress. Just used noose, anklestraps and handcuffs. . ."

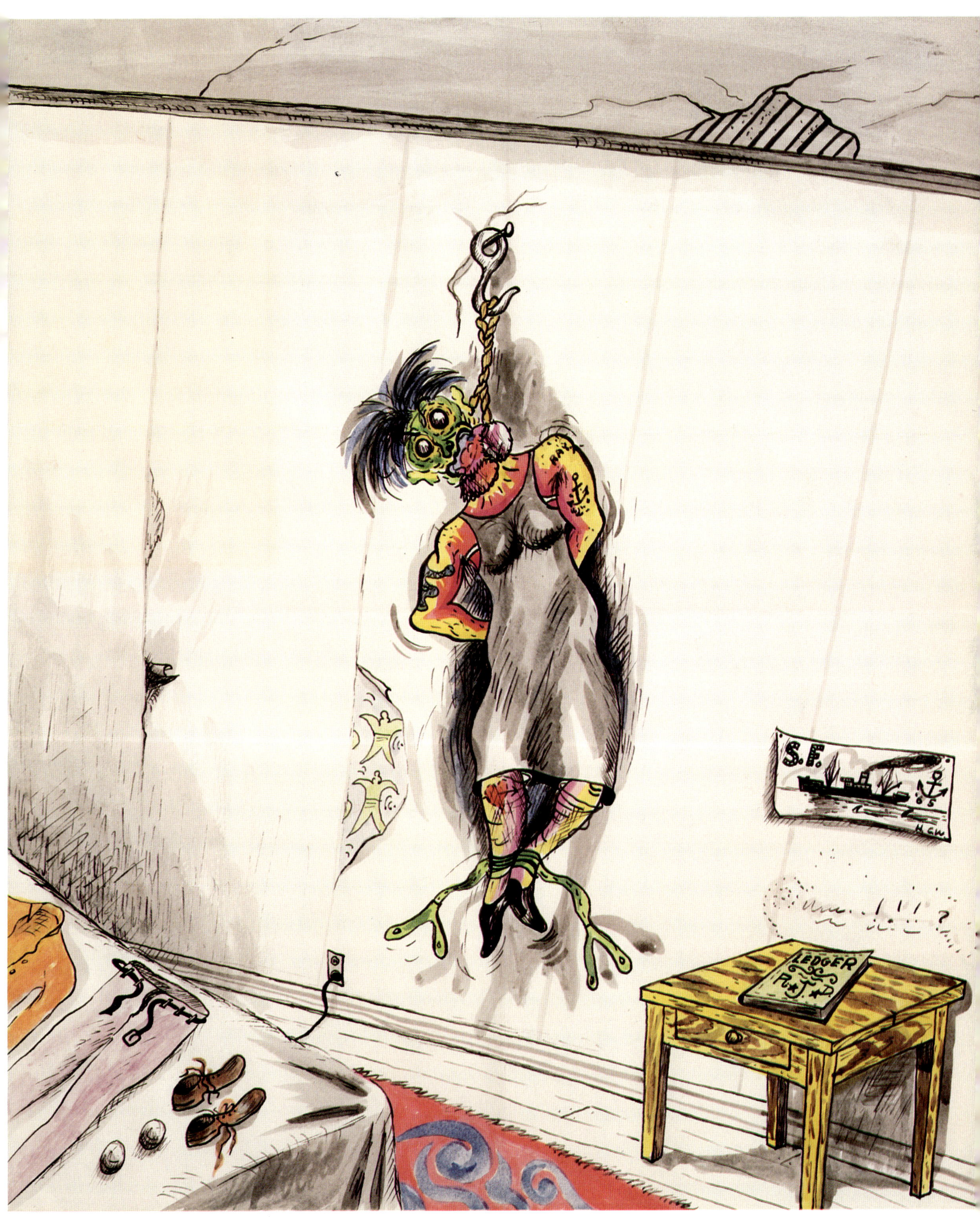
S.F.
LEDGER

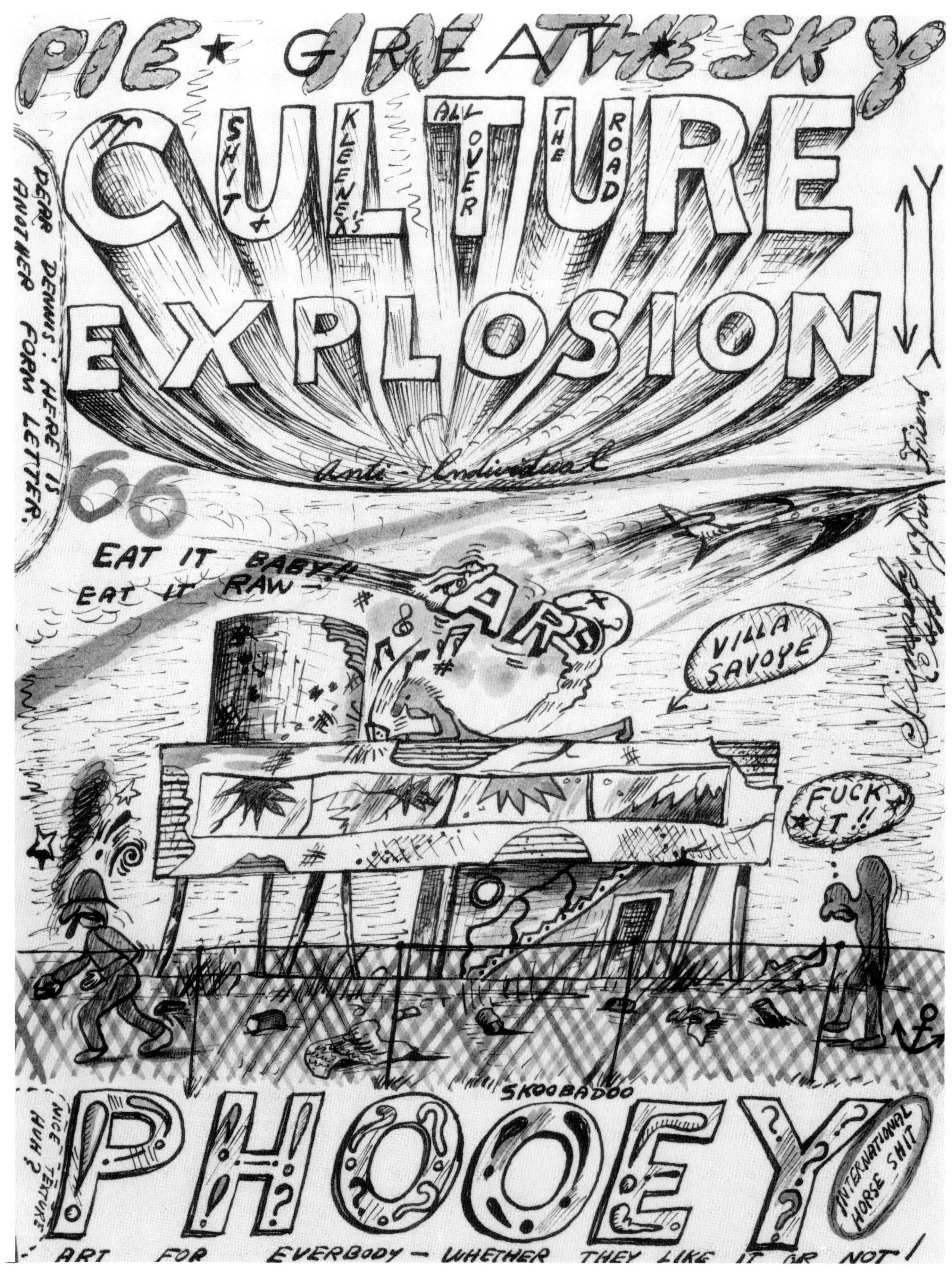

SHIT + KLEENEX'S ALL OVER THE ROAD
CULTURE
EXPLOSION
DEAR DENNIS: HERE IS ANOTHER FORM LETTER.
Anti-Individual
66
EAT IT BABY!!
EAT IT RAW
ART
VILLA SAVOYE
FUCK IT!!
SKOOBADOO
PHOOEY
INTERNATIONAL HORSE SHIT
NICE TEXTURE HUH?
ART FOR EVERBODY - WHETHER THEY LIKE IT OR NOT!

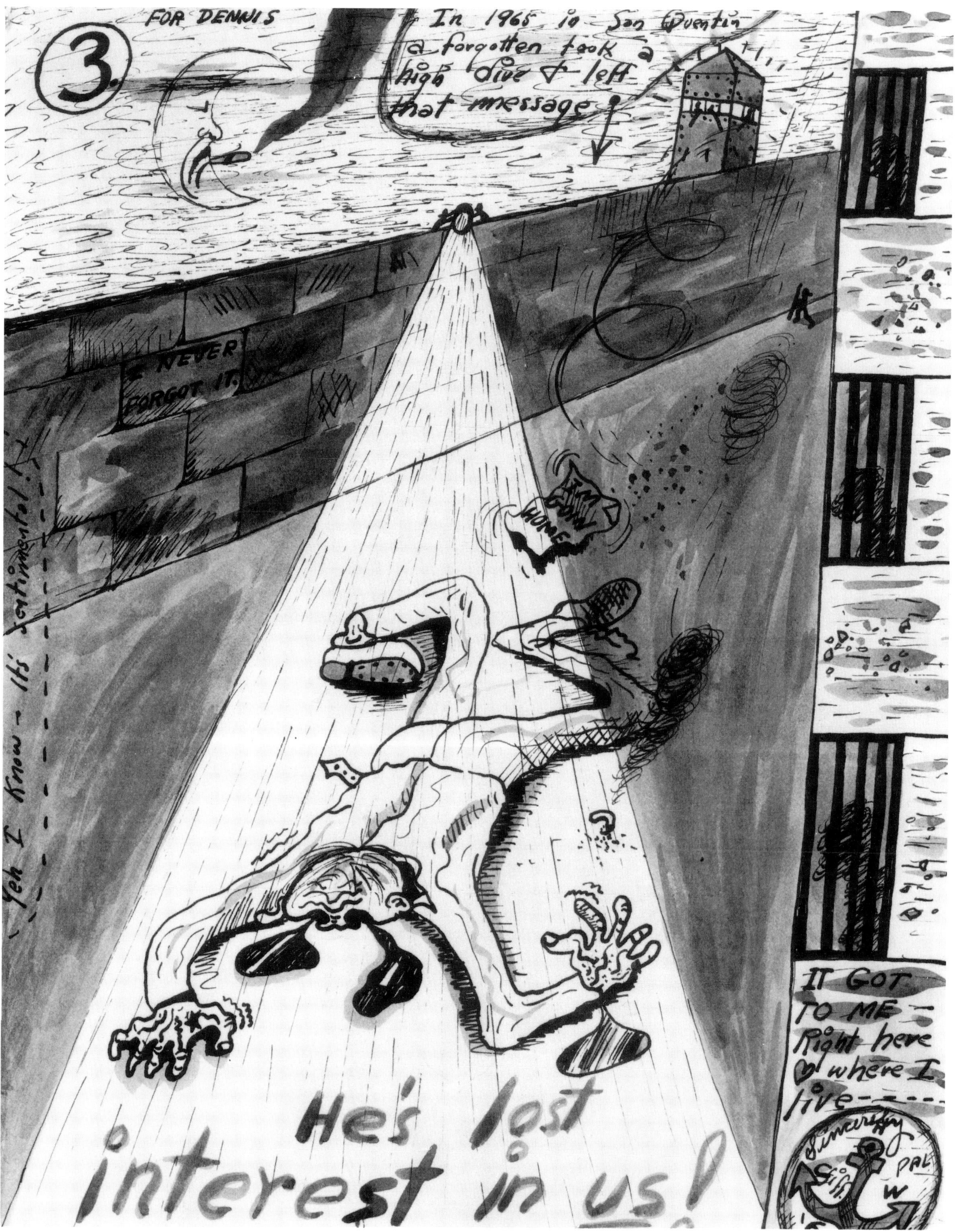

3.
FOR DENNIS
In 1965 in San Quentin a forgotten took a high dive & left that message
NEVER FORGOT IT.
Yeh I Know - It's sentimental
IT GOT TO ME - Right here where I live----
He's lost interest in us!

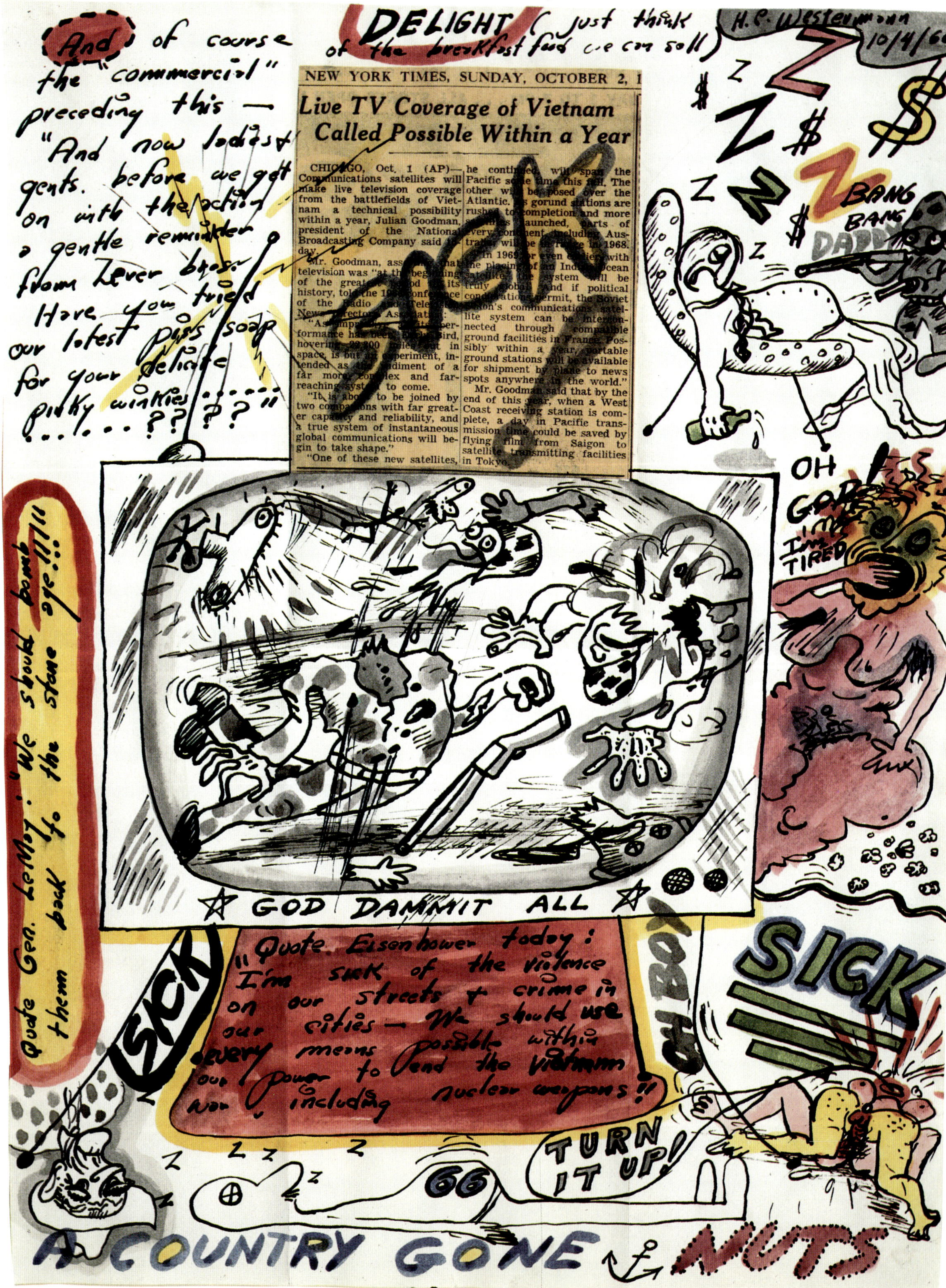

NEW YORK TIMES, SUNDAY, OCTOBER 2, 1

Live TV Coverage of Vietnam Called Possible Within a Year

CHICAGO, Oct. 1 (AP)—Communications satellites will make live television coverage from the battlefields of Vietnam a technical possibility within a year, Julian Goodman, president of the National Broadcasting Company said today.

Mr. Goodman, ass[illegible] that television was "at th[illegible] beg[illegible]ing of the great[illegible] [illegible]od [illegible] its history, told the 19[illegible] conference of the Radio [illegible] Tele[illegible] News Directors Association:

"As [illegible] [illegible] performance has been, Early Bird, hovering 22,300 miles out in space, is but an experiment, intended as [illegible] rudiment of a far more complex and far-reaching system to come.

"It is about to be joined by two companions with far greater capacity and reliability, and a true system of instantaneous global communications will begin to take shape."

"One of these new satellites," he continued, "will span the Pacific some time this fall. The other will be posed over the Atlantic. As gorund stations are rushed to completion and more [illegible] launched, parts of every continent, including Australia, will be in [illegible] in 1968.

"In 1969 or even earlier with the placing of an Indian Ocean satellite, the system will be truly global. And if political considerations permit, the Soviet Union's communications satellite system can be interconnected through compatible ground facilities in France. Possibly within a year, portable ground stations will be available for shipment by plane to news spots anywhere in the world."

Mr. Goodman said that by the end of this year, when a West Coast receiving station is complete, a day in Pacific transmission time could be saved by flying film from Saigon to satellite transmitting facilities in Tokyo.

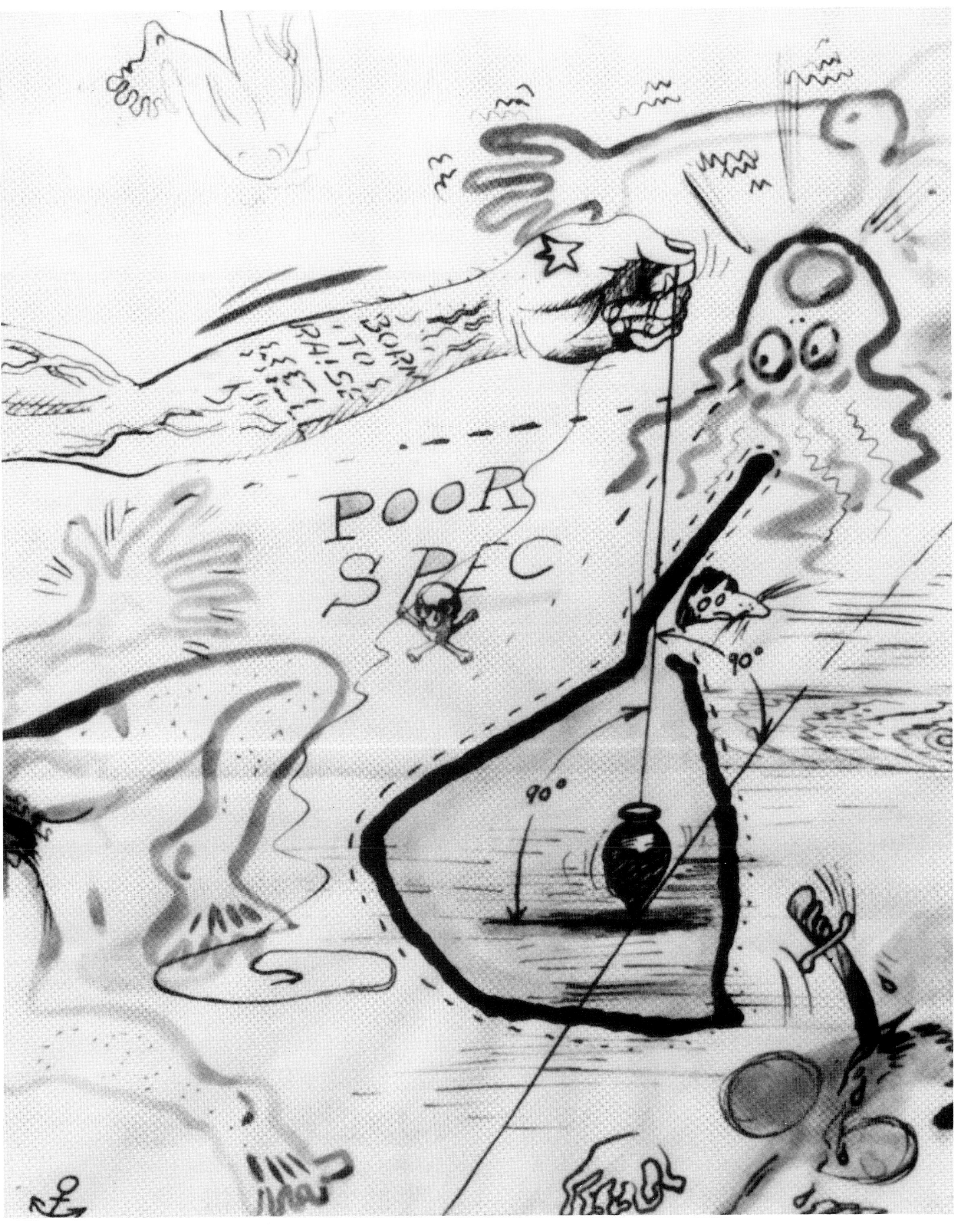
BORN TO RAISE
POOR SPEC
90°
90°

June 17, 1968

→ There are some men in this country whose job it is to just sit on their big fat pratts + drive around all day, drive around looking for beautiful examples of architecture + things — These they mark for future destruction. Well this is not my job, in fact I am the complete opposite of this.

Respectfully, H.C. Westermann

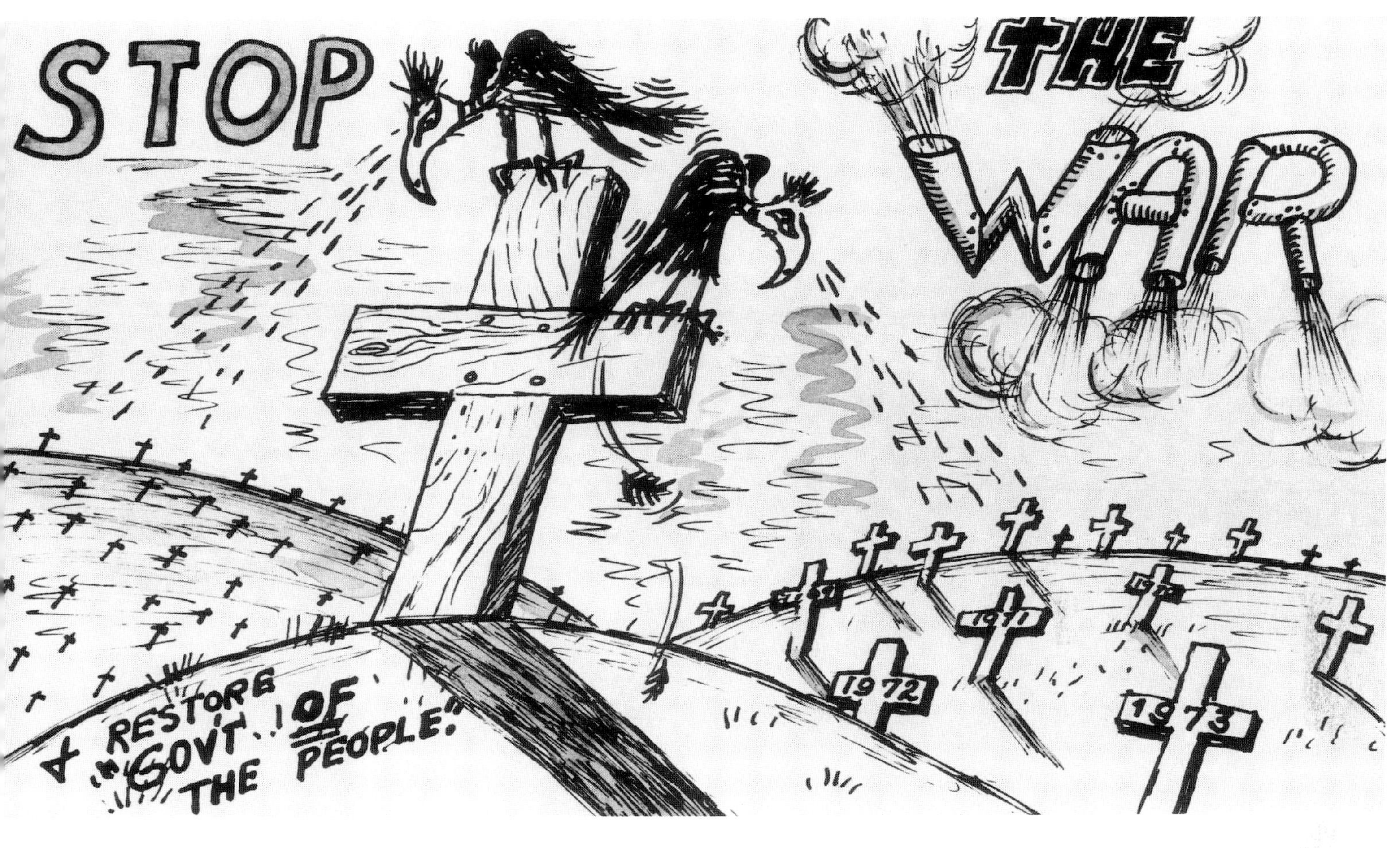

from a letter to Bruce and Doris Oxford March 29, 1978

It's a funny thing, eventually I did come around to understanding the logic of your political stand. That took years on my part. Politically, in the beginning of our friendship I was about the dumbest fucker that ever lived, really a simpleton + of course I can see that now. But then I had no exposure except from that archaic L.A. + the fascistic Marine Corps. That was all I knew + I'm ashamed of myself for being that idiotic! But I learned thanks to great people like yourself, etc. + just putting my time in. You'd be surprised now how I "piss and moan" + rant + rave about just everything at this stage of the game. Ha, ha, ha, + that includes all clubs, bureaucracies, institutions, conventions, all governments, gallery dealers, professors, the whole mother fucking works. That's sort of terrible isn't it (+ oh yeh, all politicians). I guess I'm really some kind of fucking nut!

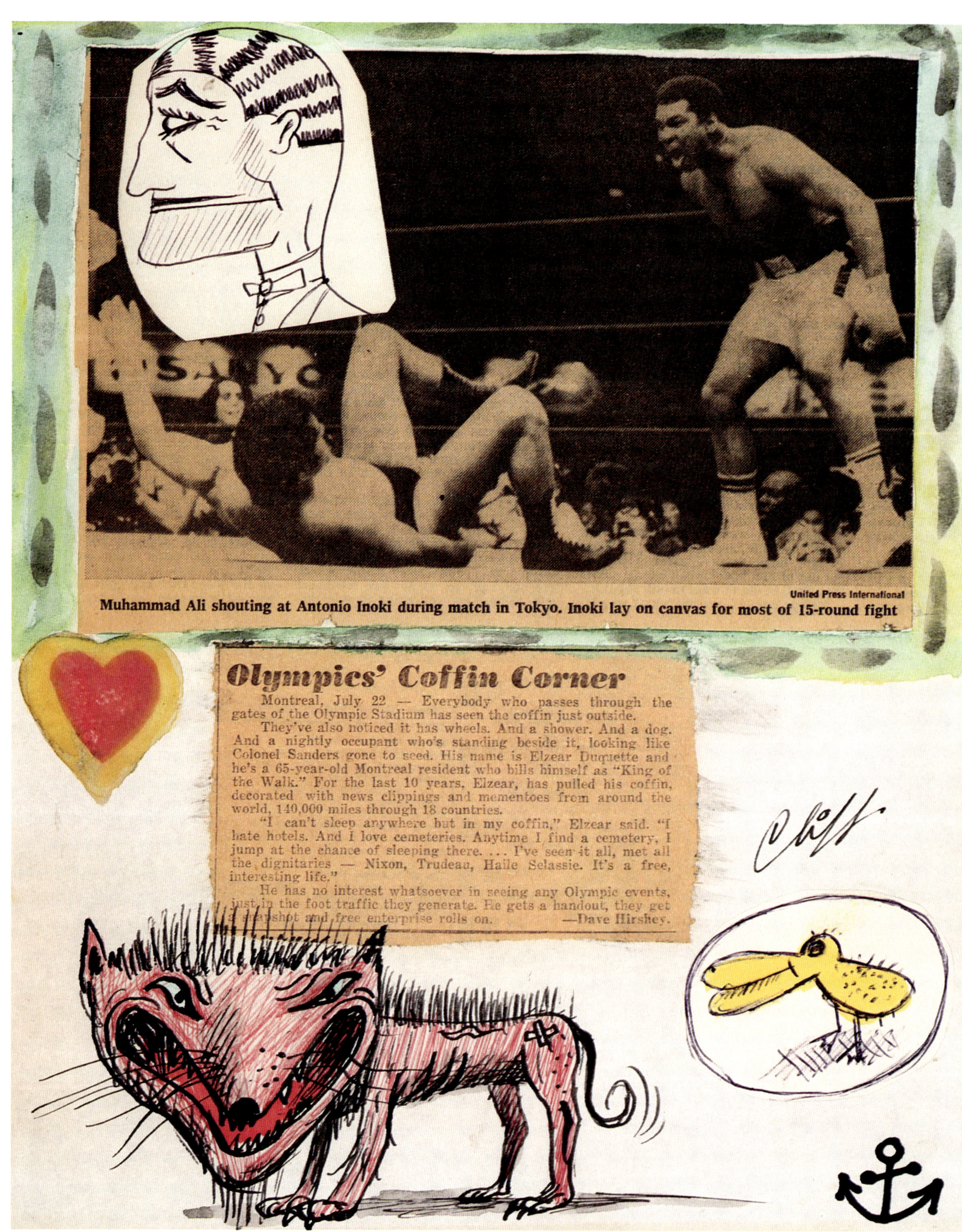

Muhammad Ali shouting at Antonio Inoki during match in Tokyo. Inoki lay on canvas for most of 15-round fight

Olympics' Coffin Corner

Montreal, July 22 — Everybody who passes through the gates of the Olympic Stadium has seen the coffin just outside.

They've also noticed it has wheels. And a shower. And a dog. And a nightly occupant who's standing beside it, looking like Colonel Sanders gone to seed. His name is Elzear Duquette and he's a 65-year-old Montreal resident who bills himself as "King of the Walk." For the last 10 years, Elzear, has pulled his coffin, decorated with news clippings and mementoes from around the world, 140,000 miles through 18 countries.

"I can't sleep anywhere but in my coffin," Elzear said. "I hate hotels. And I love cemeteries. Anytime I find a cemetery, I jump at the chance of sleeping there. ... I've seen it all, met all the dignitaries — Nixon, Trudeau, Haile Selassie. It's a free, interesting life."

He has no interest whatsoever in seeing any Olympic events, just in the foot traffic they generate. He gets a handout, they get a snapshot and free enterprise rolls on. —Dave Hirshey.

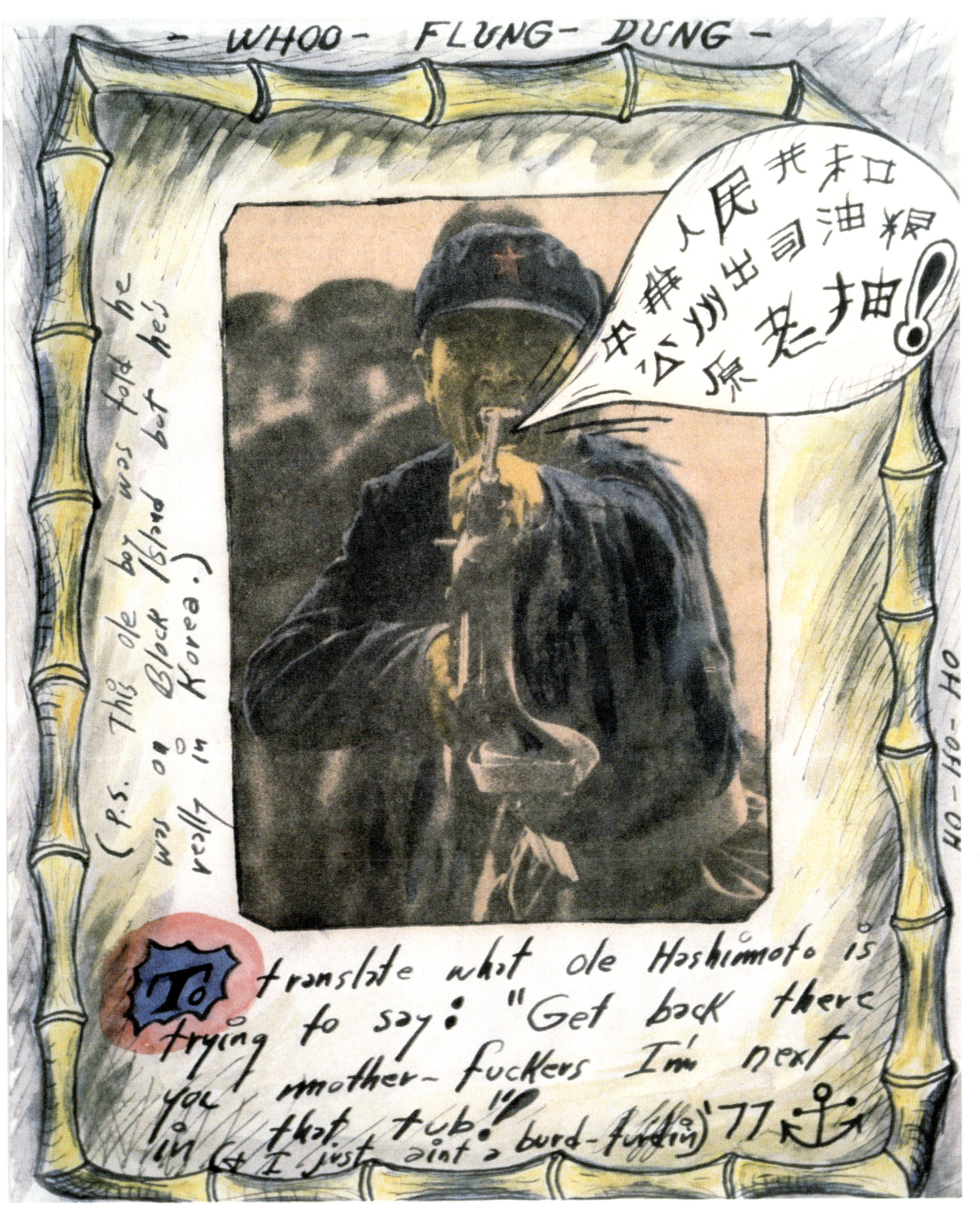
- WHOO- FLUNG- DUNG -
中華人民共和
公州出司油粮
原老抽!
(P.S. This ole boy was told he was on Black Island but he's really in Korea.)
HO-HO-HO
To translate whst ole Hashimoto is trying to say: "Get back there you motherfuckers I'm next in that tub!" (& I just aint a burd-fuckin) '77

Friends

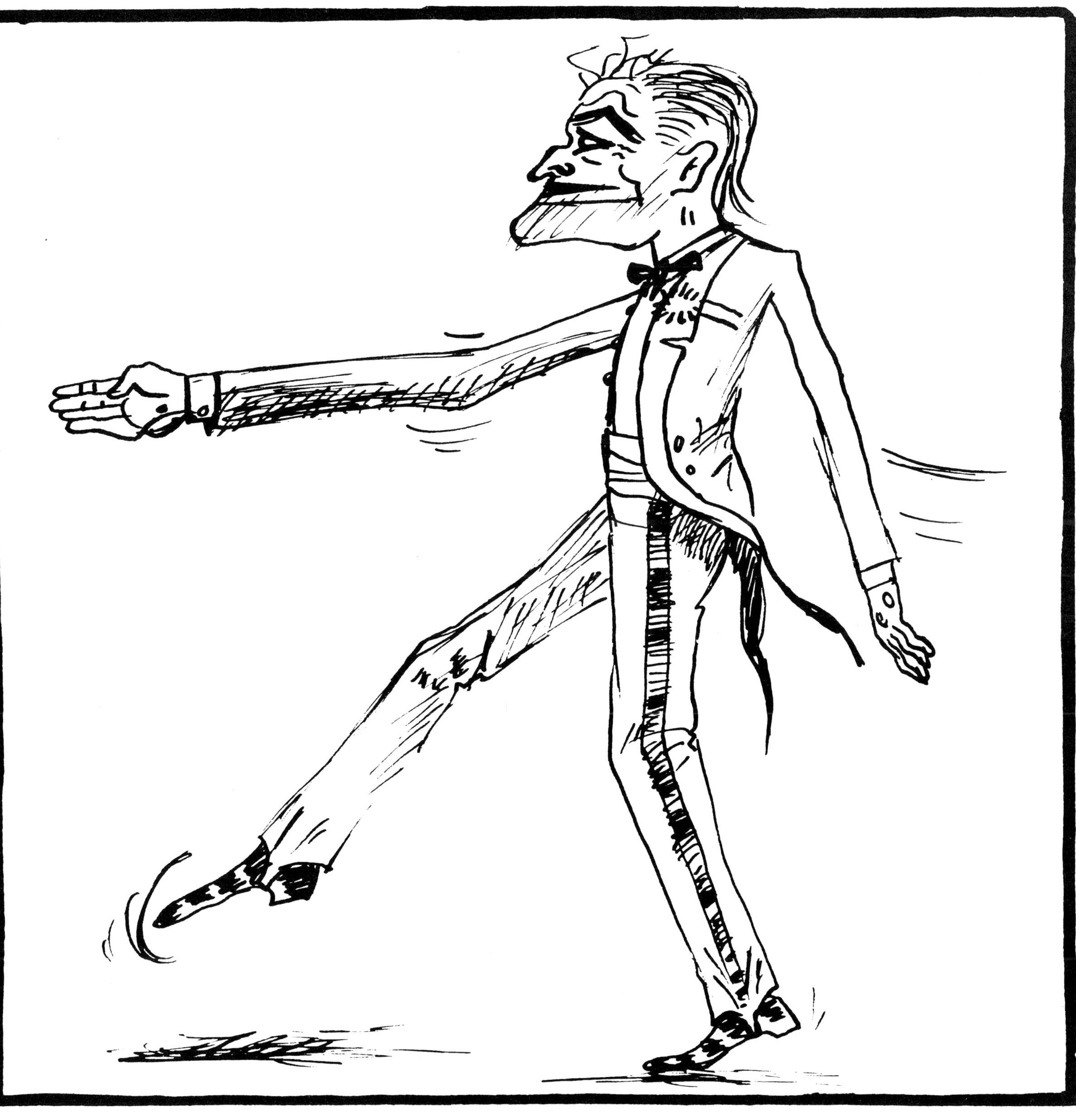

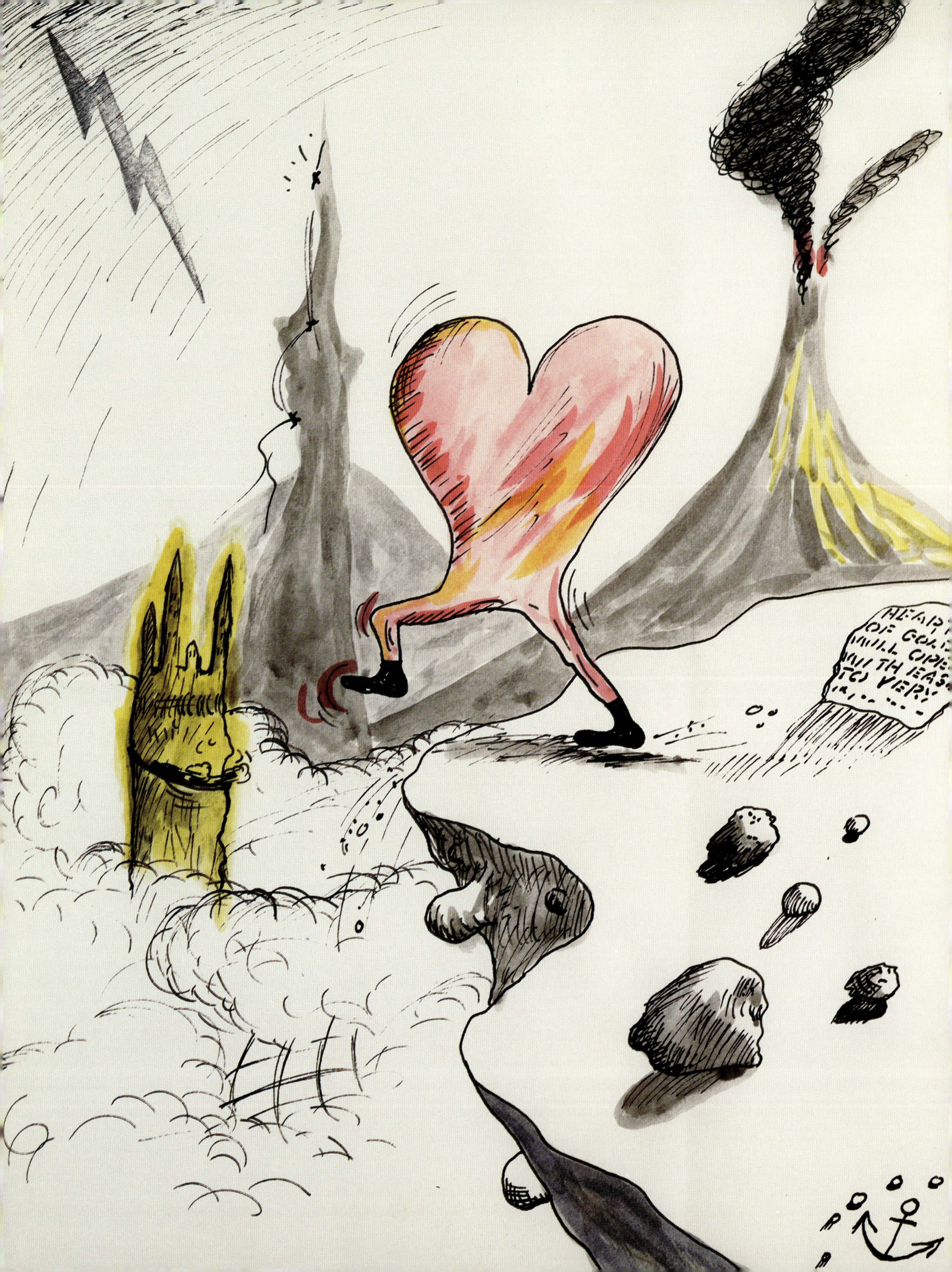
HEART
OF GOL
WILL OPE
WITH EAS
TO VERY

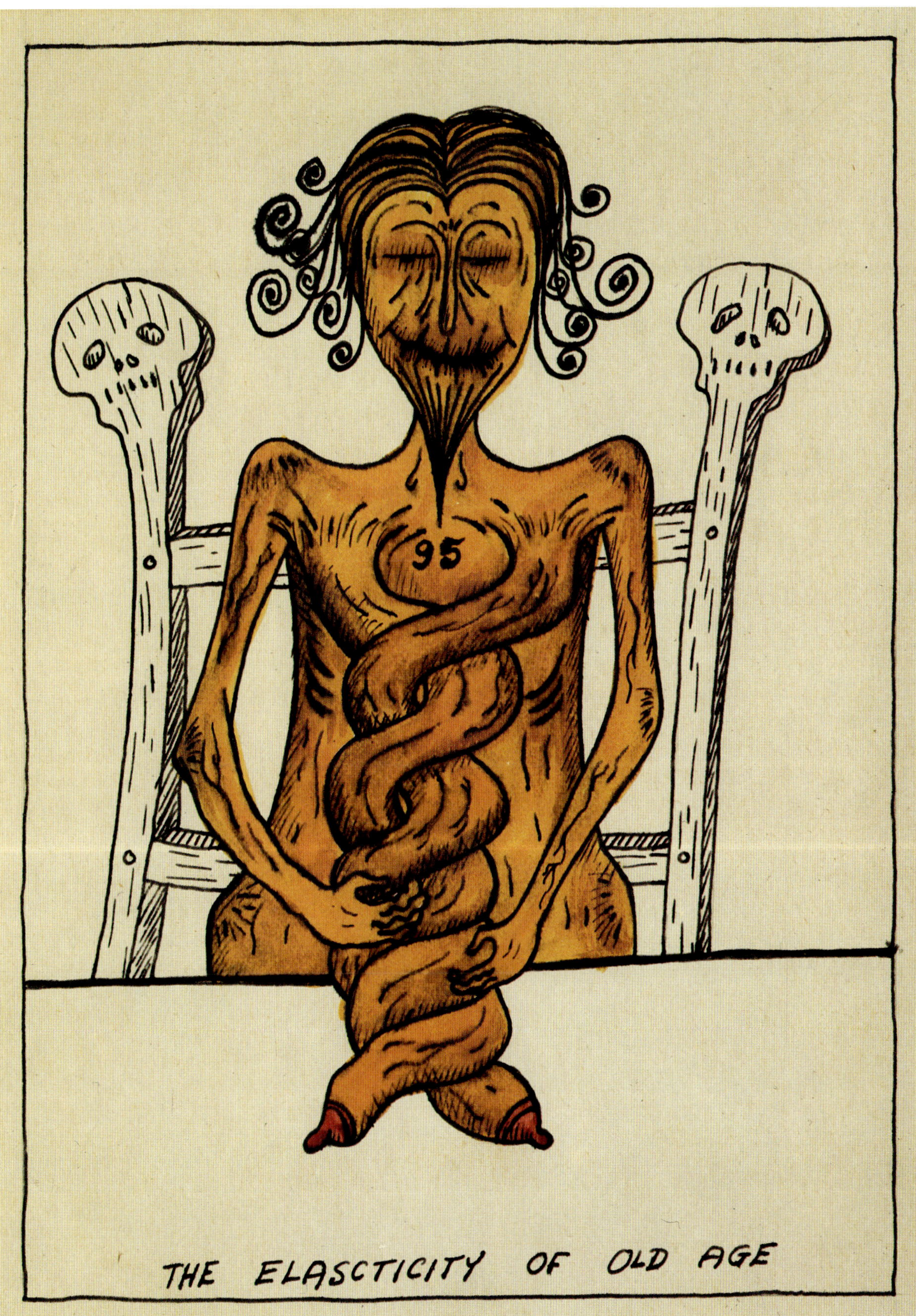
95
THE ELASCTICITY OF OLD AGE

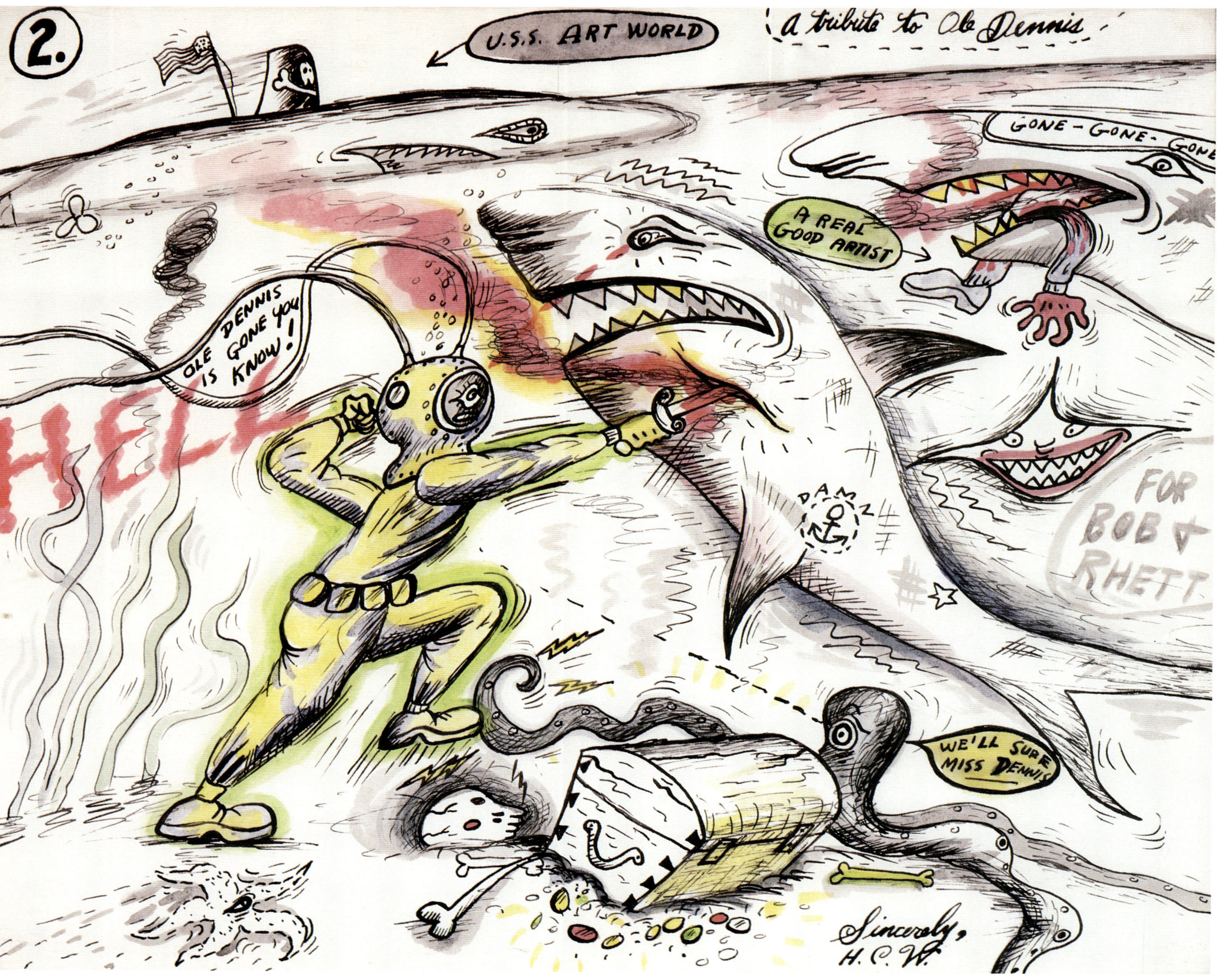

2.
U.S.S. ART WORLD
A tribute to Ole Dennis
GONE-GONE-GONE
A REAL GOOD ARTIST
OLE DENNIS GONE YOU IS KNOW!
HELL
DAMN
FOR BOB & RHETT
WE'LL SURE MISS DENNIS
Sincerely, H.C.W.

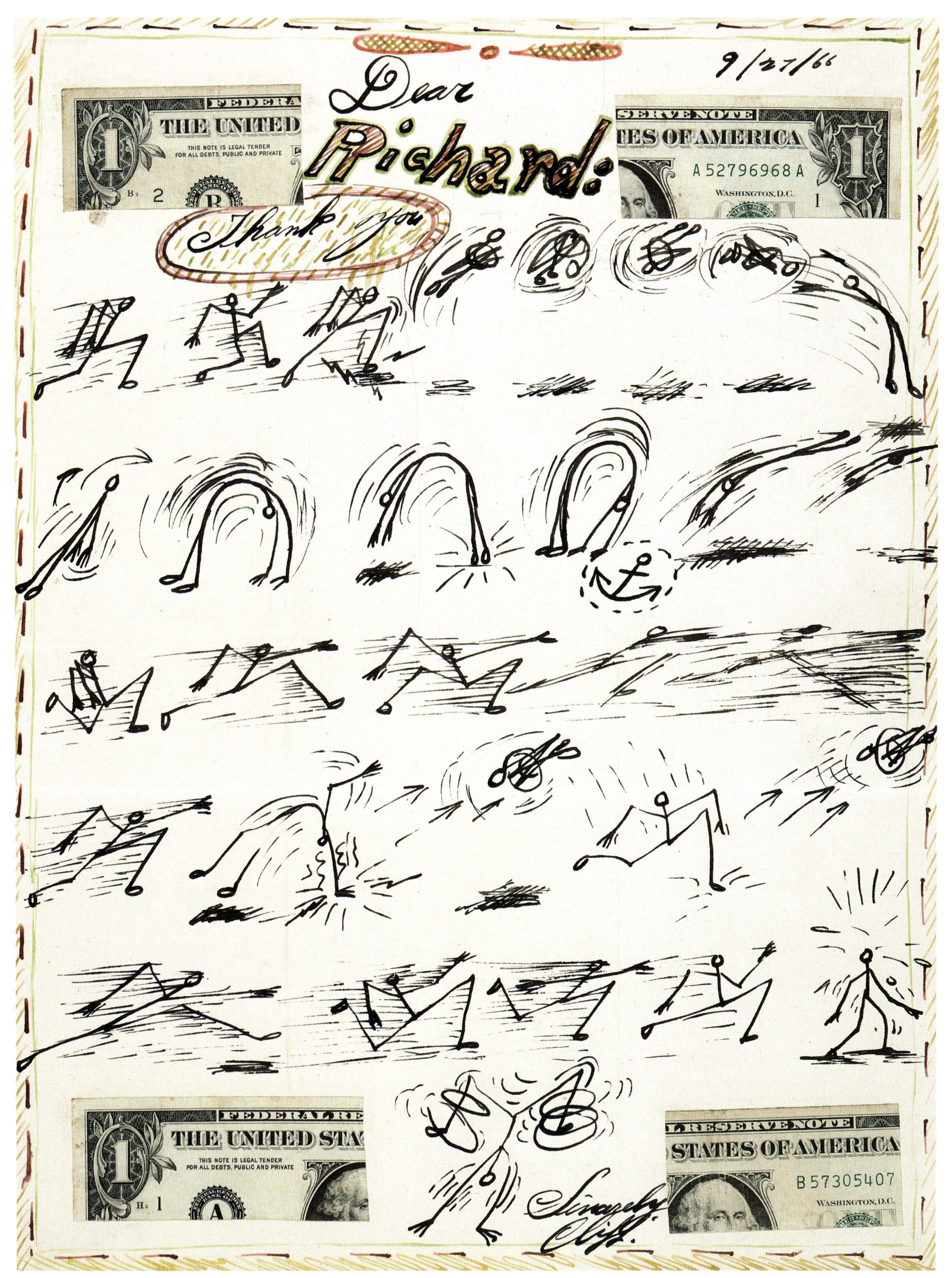
9/27/66

Dear Richard:

Thank you

Sincerely
Cliff.

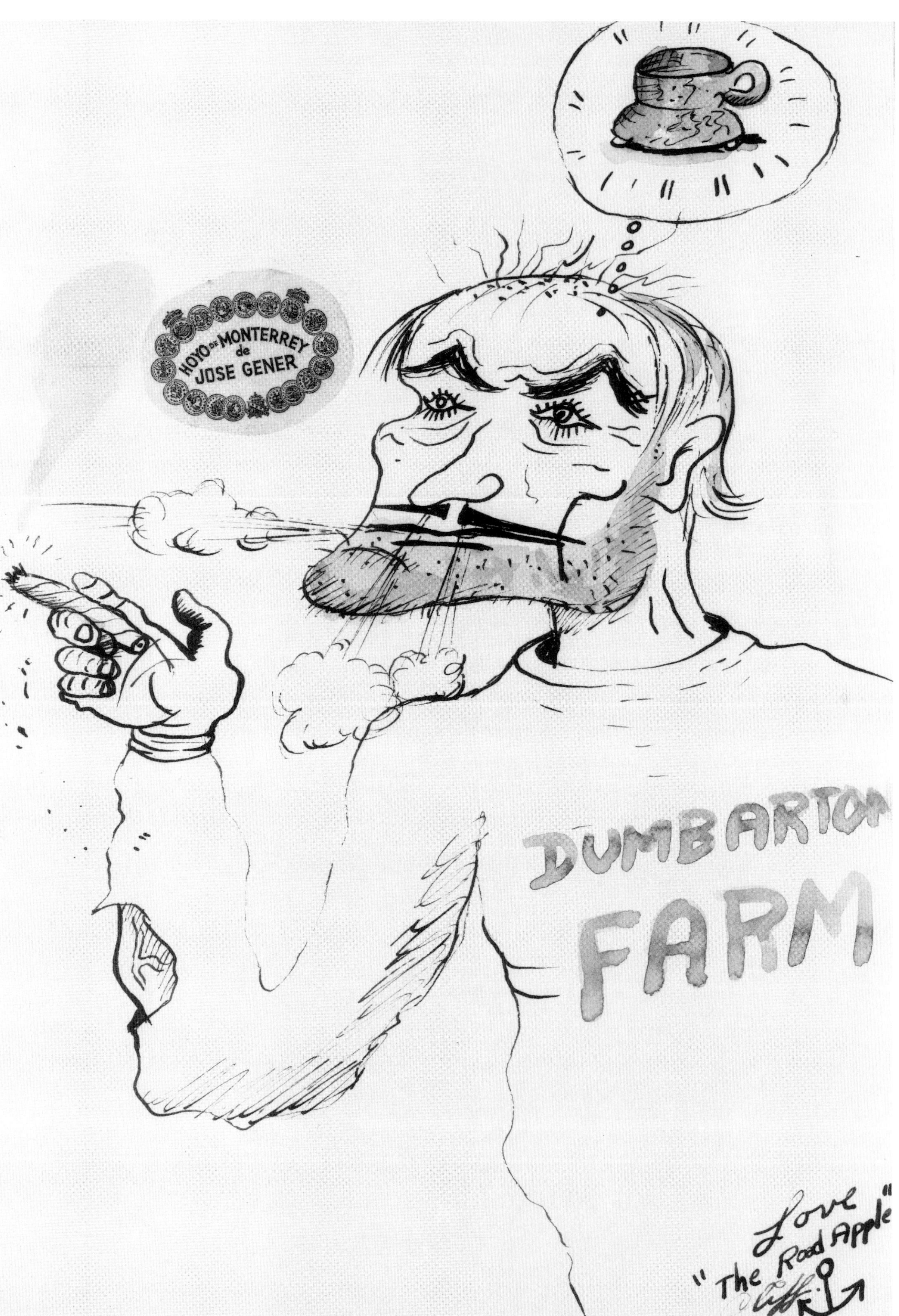
HOYO DE MONTERREY
de
JOSE GENER
DUMBARTON
FARM
Love
"The Road Apple"

DEC 6, 1968

Dear Allan:

TE-AMO is about my favorite cigar & I want to thank you very much for sending that box to me — I'm sure enjoying them. The only crisis on the plane coming back was that the stewardess ran out of paper cups. It's good to be home & I'll bet you feel the same way. Say hello to Jean & the gang.

Sincerely,

Cliff

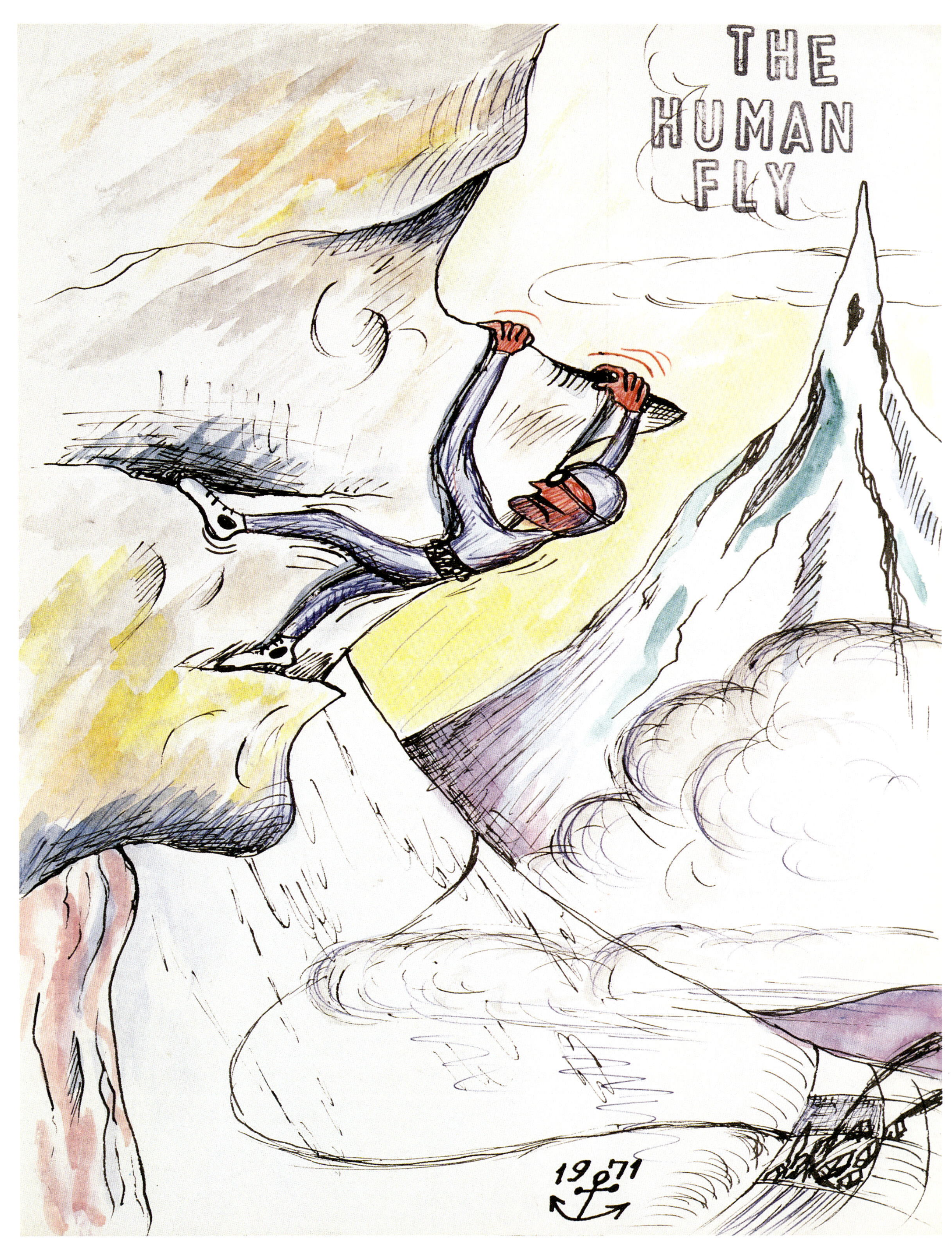
THE HUMAN FLY
1971

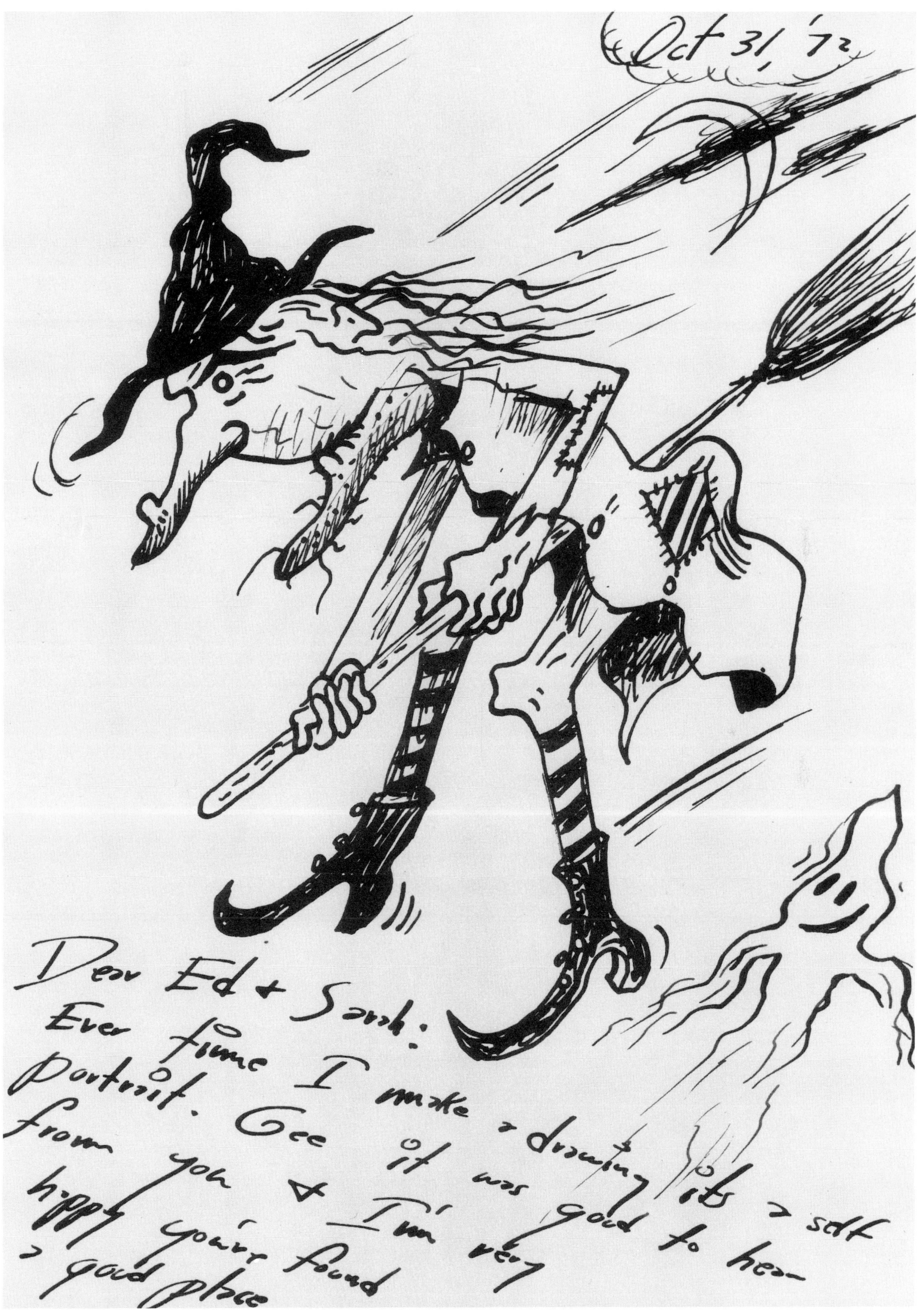
Oct 31, '72
Dear Ed + Sarah:
Ever time I make a drawing its a self
portrait. Gee it was good to hear
from you + I'm very
happy you've found
a good place

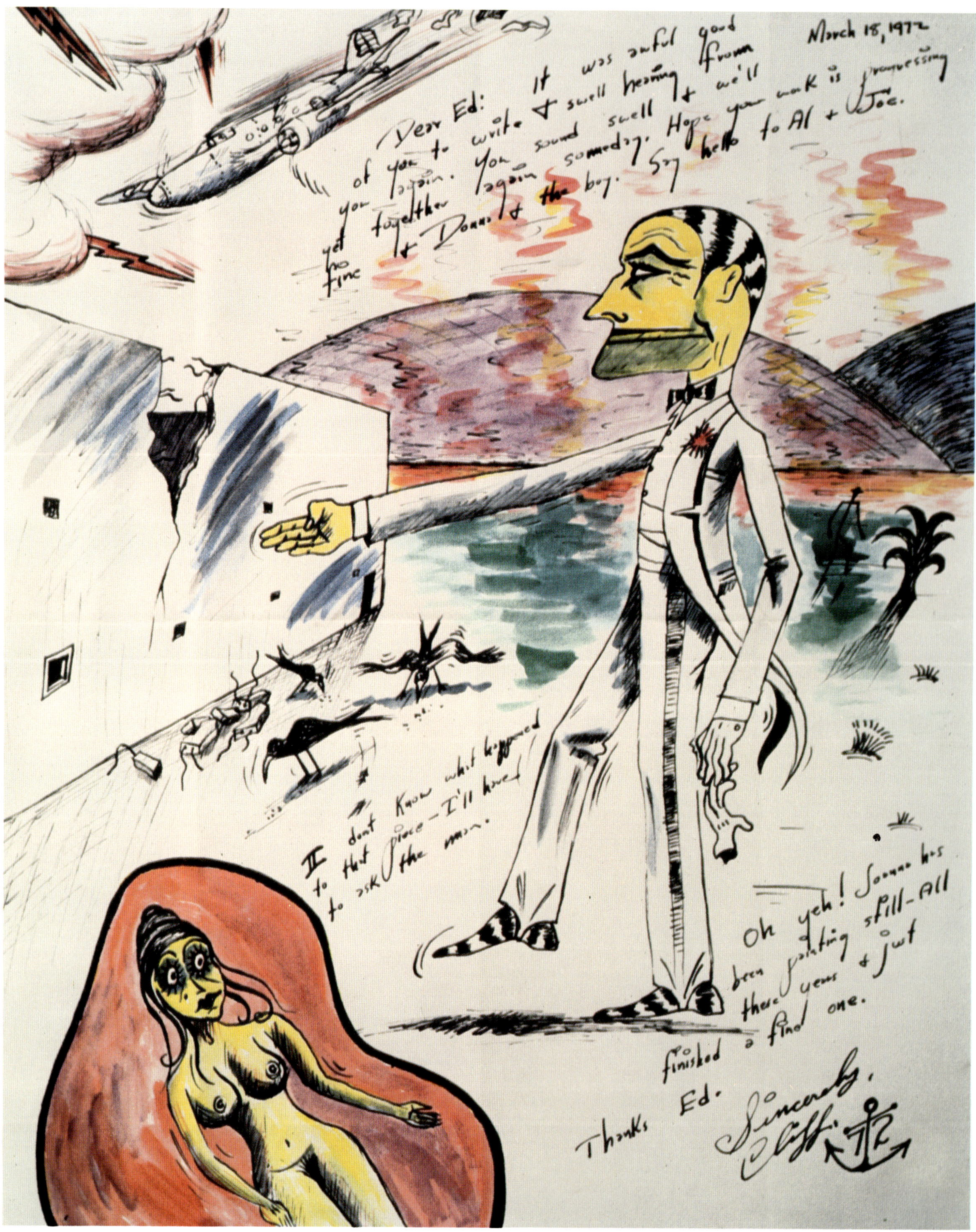

March 18, 1972
Dear Ed: It was awful good of you to write & swell hearing from you again. You sound swell & we'll get together again someday. Hope your work is progressing fine & Donna & the boy. Say hello to Al & Joe.
I don't know what happened to that piece — I'll have to ask the man.
Oh yeh! Donna has been painting still-All these years & just finished a fine one.
Thanks Ed.
Sincerely, Cliff

Nov. 2, 1972

Dear Al:

We went to a party the other & there were a bunch of real flying ass-holes there. I got sick- bad- & threw up like #1 & as my teeth went out with all the junk I snapped them right out of thin air & shoved them back in my fuckin head, like #2. It took me a week to get over that one. The little woman & I have finished framing our house & are just finishing up the shingling. Yeh Al - The little woman gets right up there with me & we chug a lug.

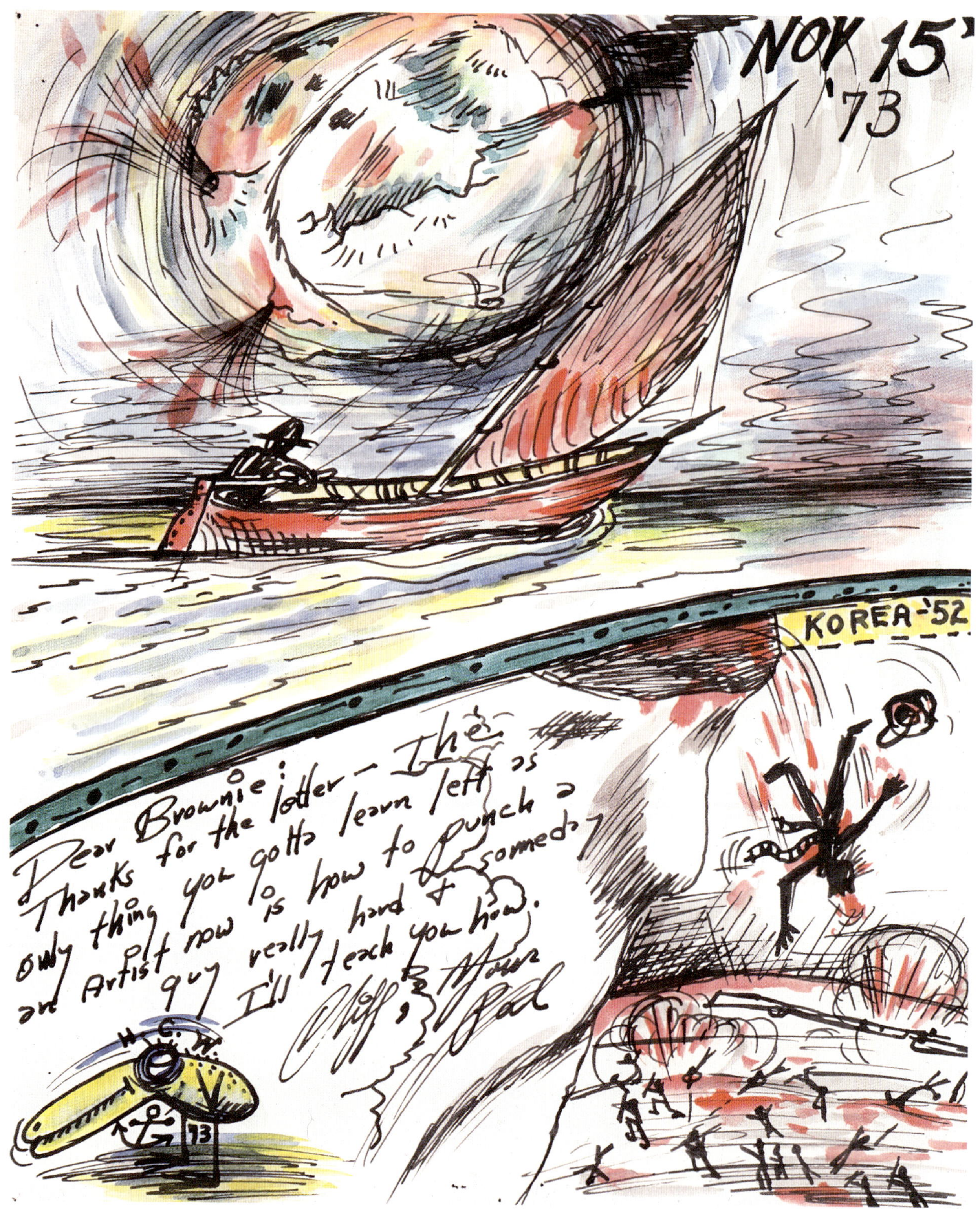

from a letter to Roger Brouard Summer, 1981

... if you want to belt him one all you have to do is smack him in the nose (remember that) — hard + fast. As soon as he sees the blood, you'll have it made + it hurts a little too to get smacked in the nose. The blood is the secret, that and hitting first! That takes the fight right out of any mother-fucker. That's my big secret kid + it won't cost you a nickel for the instruction.

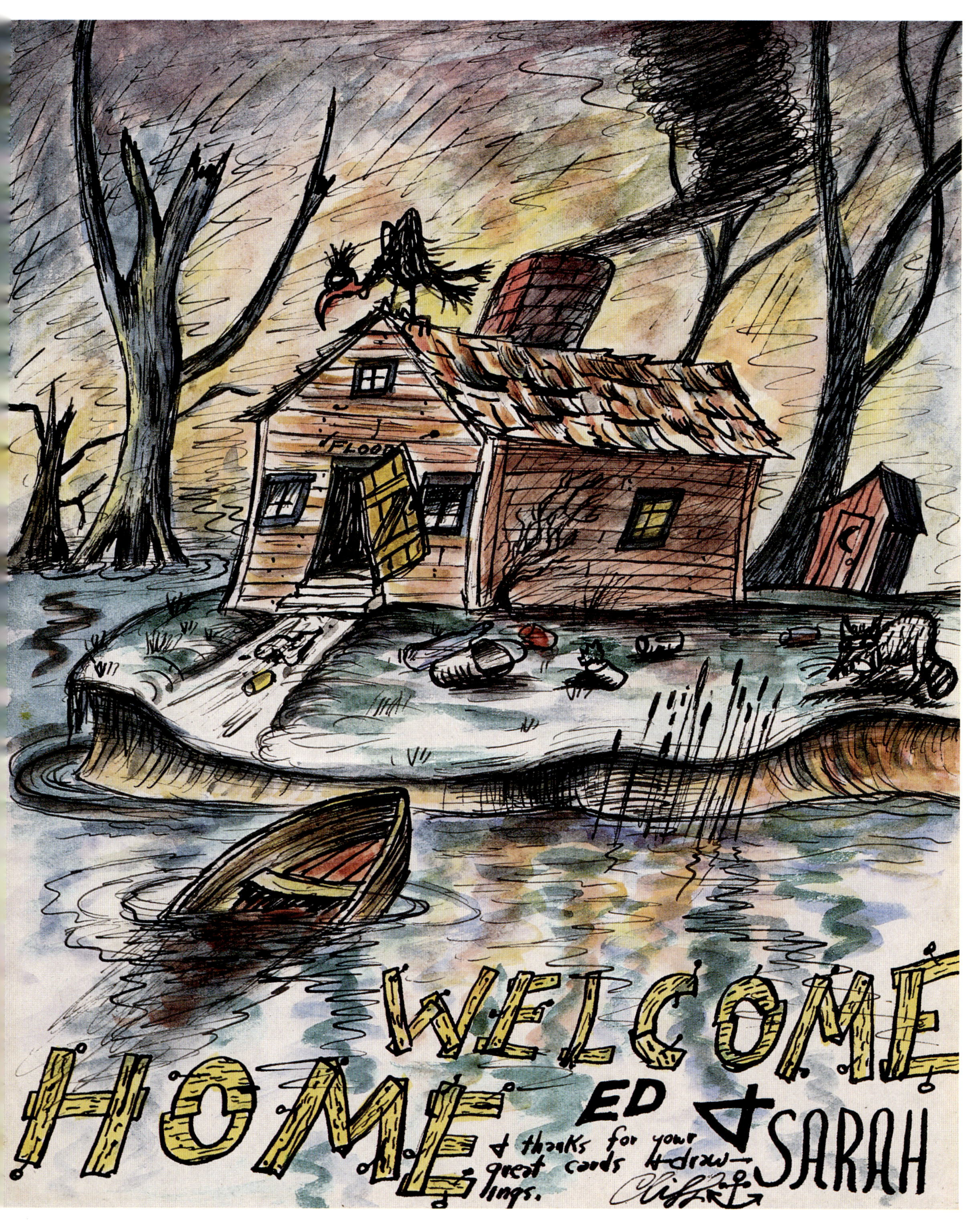
FLOO
WELCOME
HOME
ED & SARAH
& thanks for your great cards & drawings.
Cliff

September 4, 1974

Dear Dr. Laragh:

I was formerly a patient of Dr. Brunner + I assume soon of Dr. Case (I have an appointment with him on Sept 12). I have been a patient about 2 years now + have undergone the series of pills + drugs (aldactone, inderol, diuril, serposil, etc): I have had excellent general health for years but these treatments seem to undermine the fact. They seem to have an adverse effect upon my general well being + I have thrown up a lot, had violent stomach aches, etc. Last January I entered the hospital for the three weeks of tests etc. It was a long three weeks + when I left I didn't learn anything specific or that I thought was constructive to my case. After I left I was started on another pill program: serposil, inderol + aldactone. After 2 months of feeling from bad to worse I went into a terrific tailspin — + reached the lowest depths of depression + out of desperation I went to a shrink in N.Y. + he immediately took me off serposil + put me on a program of tofrinol (an anti-dep.) of course an aftermath of the depression was the fact that this rendered me unfunctional + I have not yet been able to return to my work — however I do feel better now + quit taking the aldactone + inderol + diuril. This all started now about 3½ months ago. The tofrinol did get me over the horrible depression but I still can't do anything yet. The whole thing seems like a nightmare now. I'm trying to explain my dilemma to you sir. Naturally I don't look forward to another two years of this torture + expense. I guess I need some kind of reassurance that your program is positive + that I am not just a statistic but a real human being — it seems so impersonal somehow! I liked Dr. Brunner + I don't blame him or you or the hospital, but it is really frustrating + at times painful.

Respectfully yours,
H.C. Westermann

P.S. I would appreciate very much some sort of response to this letter. Thank you.

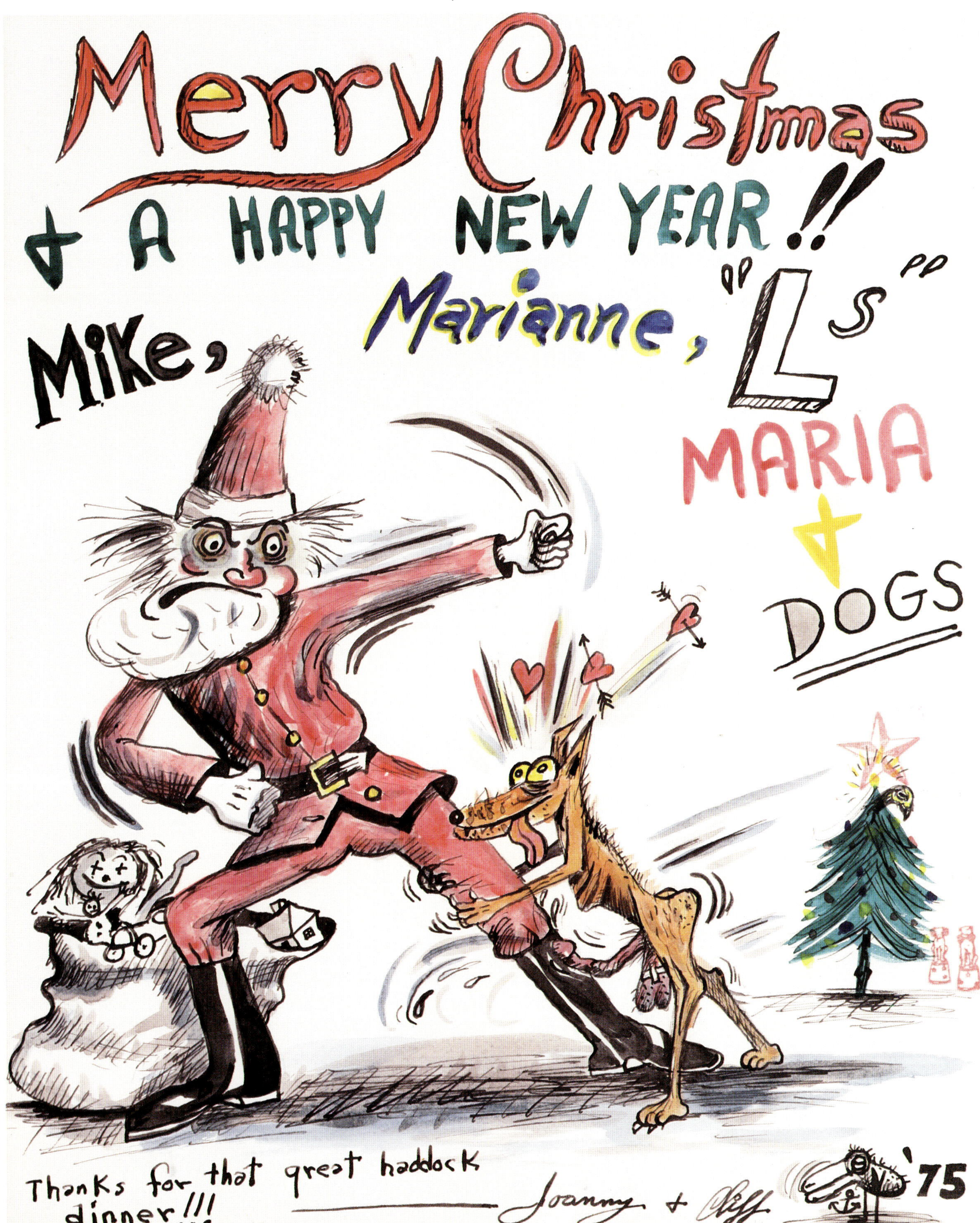
Merry Christmas
+ A HAPPY NEW YEAR!!
Mike, Marianne, "L's"
MARIA
+
DOGS
Thanks for that great haddock dinner!!!
Joanny + Cliff
'75

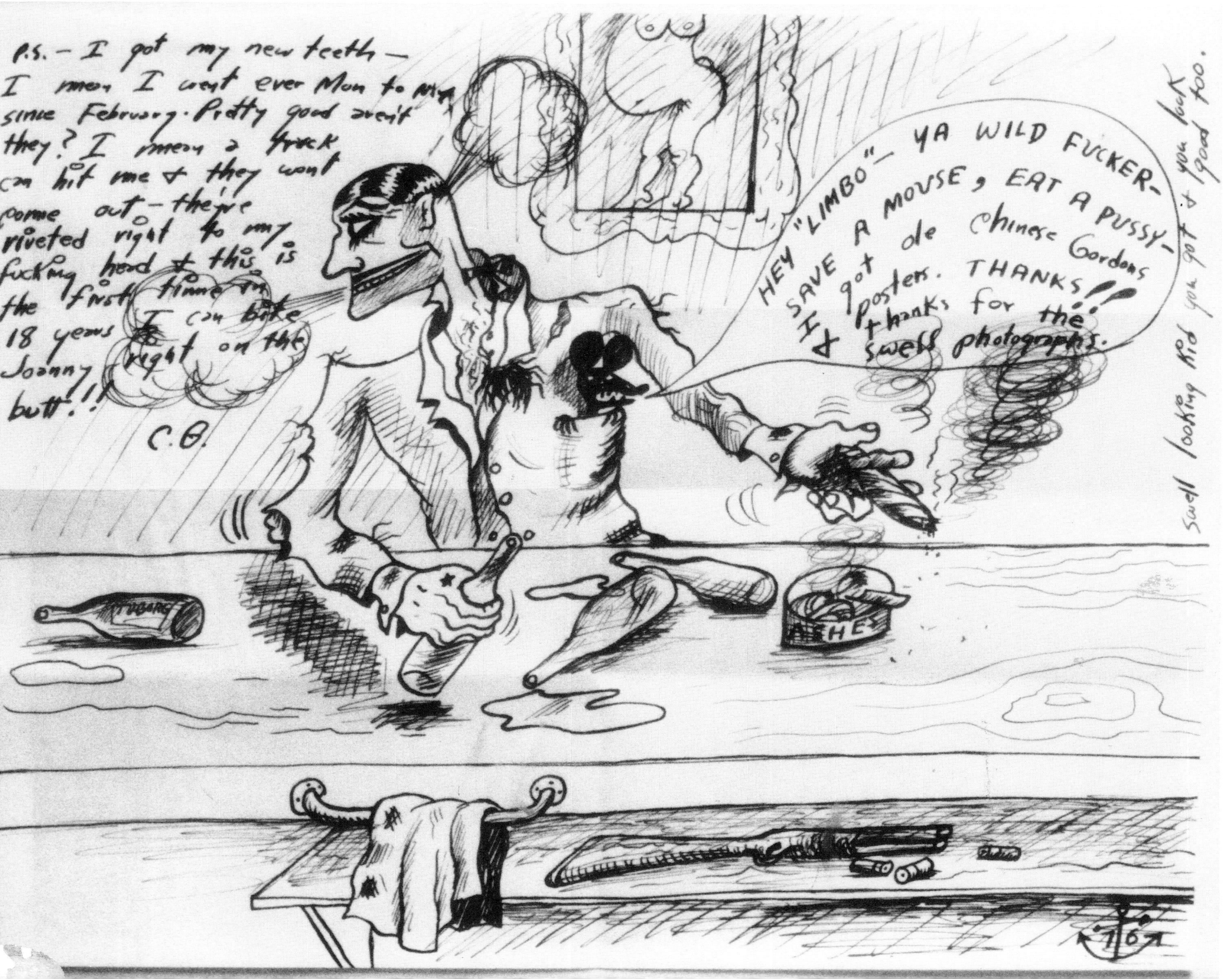
P.S. – I got my new teeth –
I mean I went ever Mon to
since February. Pretty good aren't
they? I mean a truck
can hit me & they won't
come out – they're
riveted right to my
fucking head & this is
the first time in
18 years I can bite
right on the
Joanny butt!!
C.B.
HEY "LIMBO" – YA WILD FUCKER –
SAVE A MOUSE, EAT A PUSSY –
I got de Chinese Gordons
posters. THANKS!!
& thanks for the
swell photographs.
ASHES
Swell looking kid you got & you look
good too.

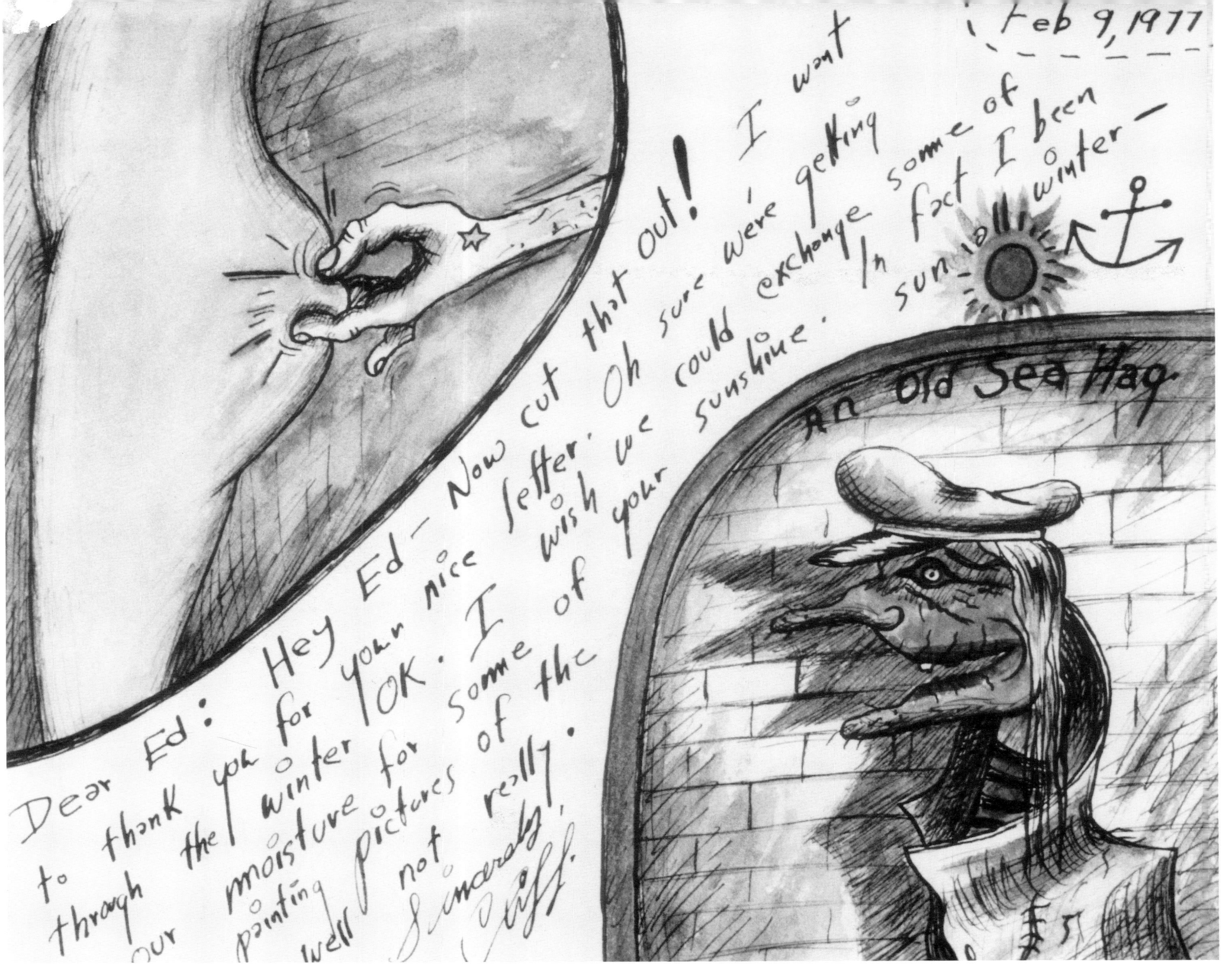
Feb 9, 1977
Dear Ed: Hey Ed— Now cut that out! I want
to thank you for your nice letter. Oh sure we're getting
through the winter OK. I wish we could exchange some of
our moisture for some of your sunshine. In fact I been
painting pictures of the sun winter—
well not really.
Sincerely,
Cliff.
An Old Sea Hag

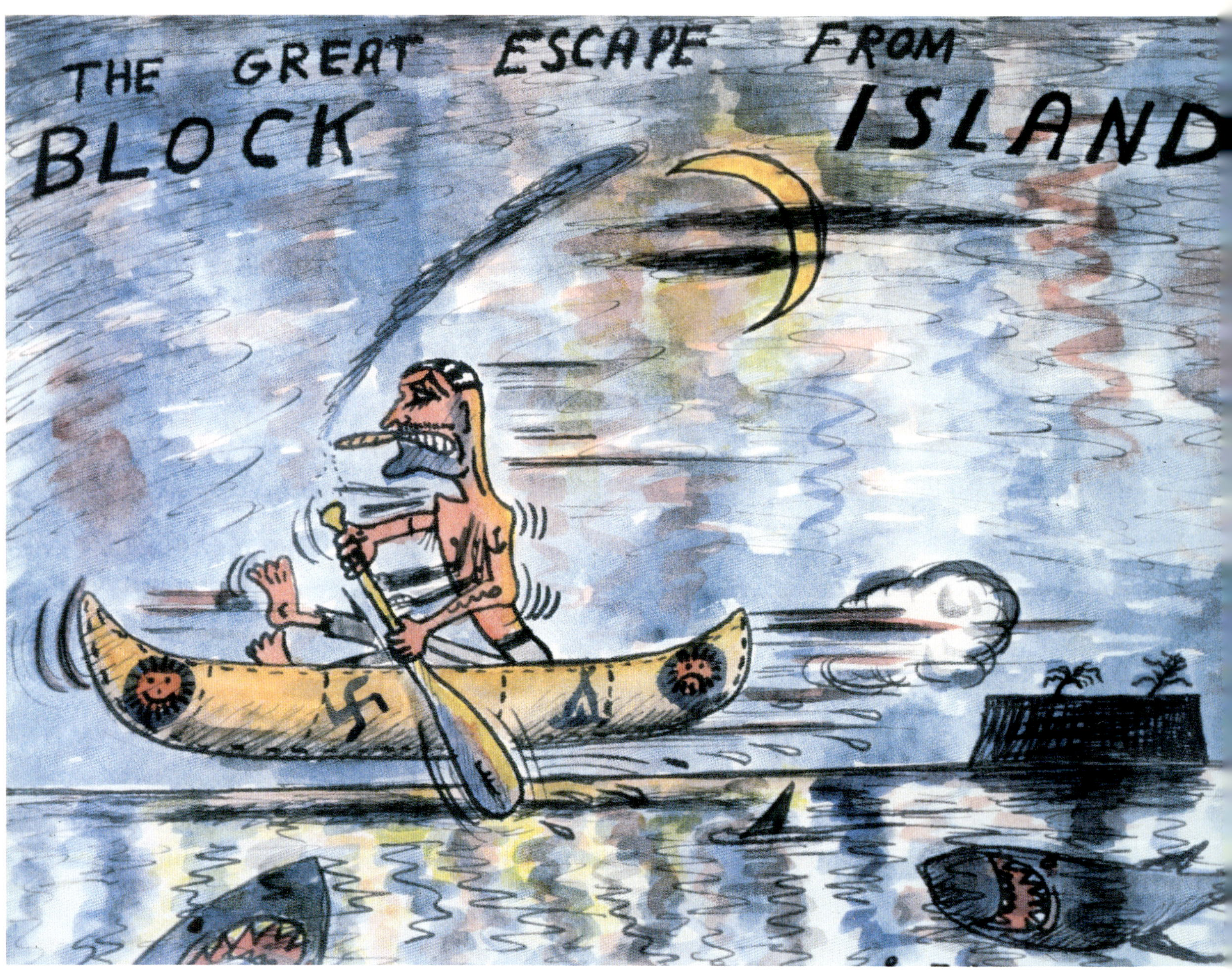

from a letter to Robert and Mavis Hudson January 4, 1978

Block Island, my ass, the next time we go on a vacation I'm going take "the little flower" to the headwaters of the Zambezi river. We'd be better off there than on that fuckin' rock. I did a sort of lecture at Rhode Island University in November (+ it is not too far from B.I.) + I started the lecture by telling them all that it was the asshole of creation etc + telling them how it came to be called B.I. (thanks to my old pal Mavis). Well they all blinked a couple of times + looked at me with "little orphan annie" eyes + I made a lot of enemies. I found out later half the faculty there + a lot of the students had summer homes on Block Island + not only that but the other half of the art dept were natives of the god-damned place. Last summer, I got a postcard from that lousy inn where we stayed cordially welcoming us back + "when would we like a reservation, blah, blah, blah" + to return the postcard post paid. I just simply put on it "you've got to be kidding" and sent it back. Why that fucker there (the mercenary bastard) wouldn't even give us a glass of water.

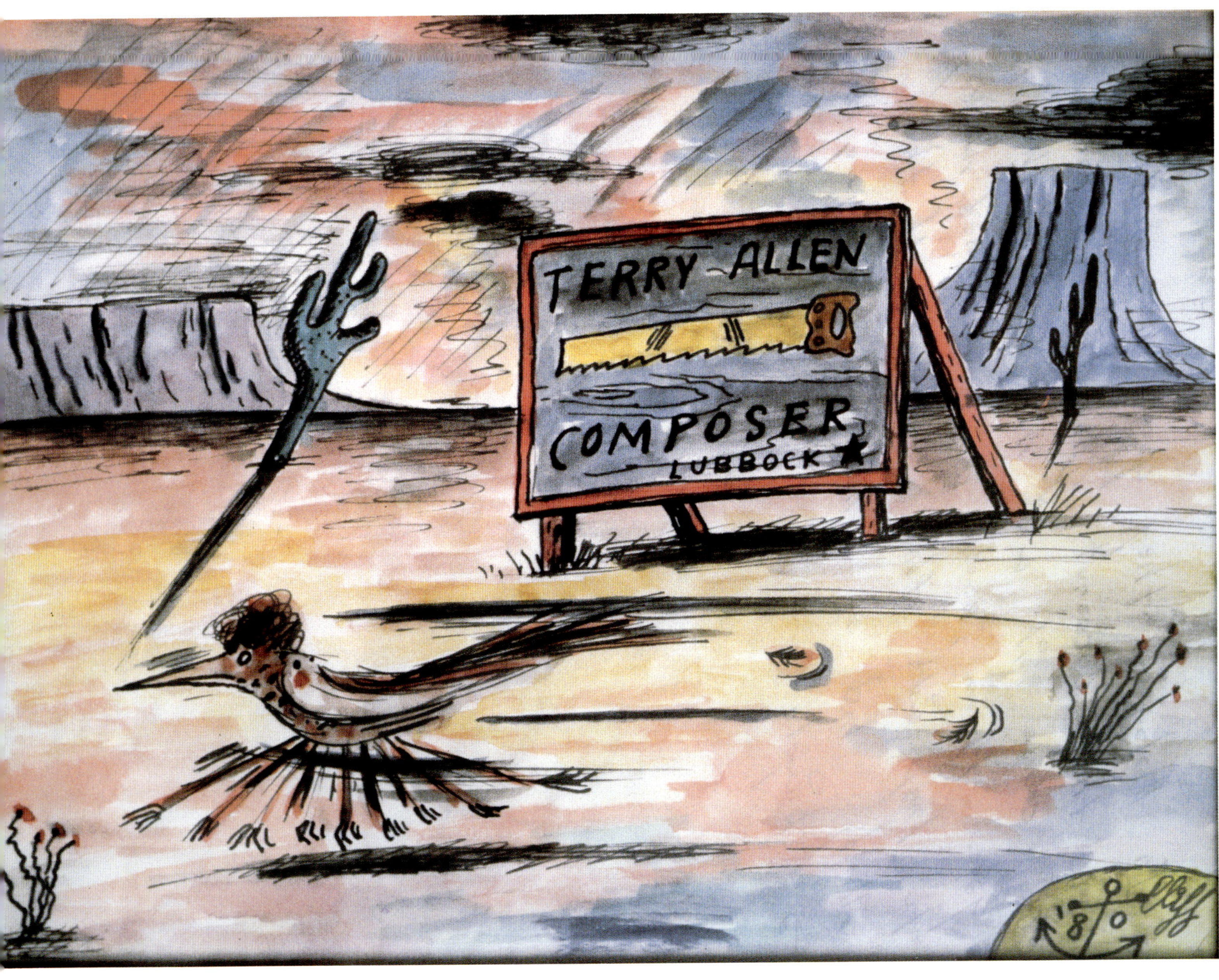

from a letter to Terry + Jo Harvey Allen June 5, 1979

Here in the East they got one country western station, in N.Y. + they play that Nashville garbage. Joanny + I once lived for a year in S.F. + I used to listen to a country western station from Oakland. At that time George Jones was living + working there + he did some really beautiful things — I really liked him. But then he got all "slicked up" + went down the drain, a long time ago + just does shit now. I don't know what happened. But your music touches me a hell of a lot more than the best of Jones + he was about the only contemporary I liked. Your music seems to be pulling against all the cheap shit that we know in this society (the destruction of beautiful architecture, the rottenness in the Govt + all the fuckin institutions for that matter, the lousy rip-offs of all the really good things + people, too, etc.) + yet, Terry, there is nothing self-righteous about your music. It's just beautiful, to me + I'll drink a "Pearl beer" (from the land of 10,000 springs — San Antonio) to that one.

Brookfield Center

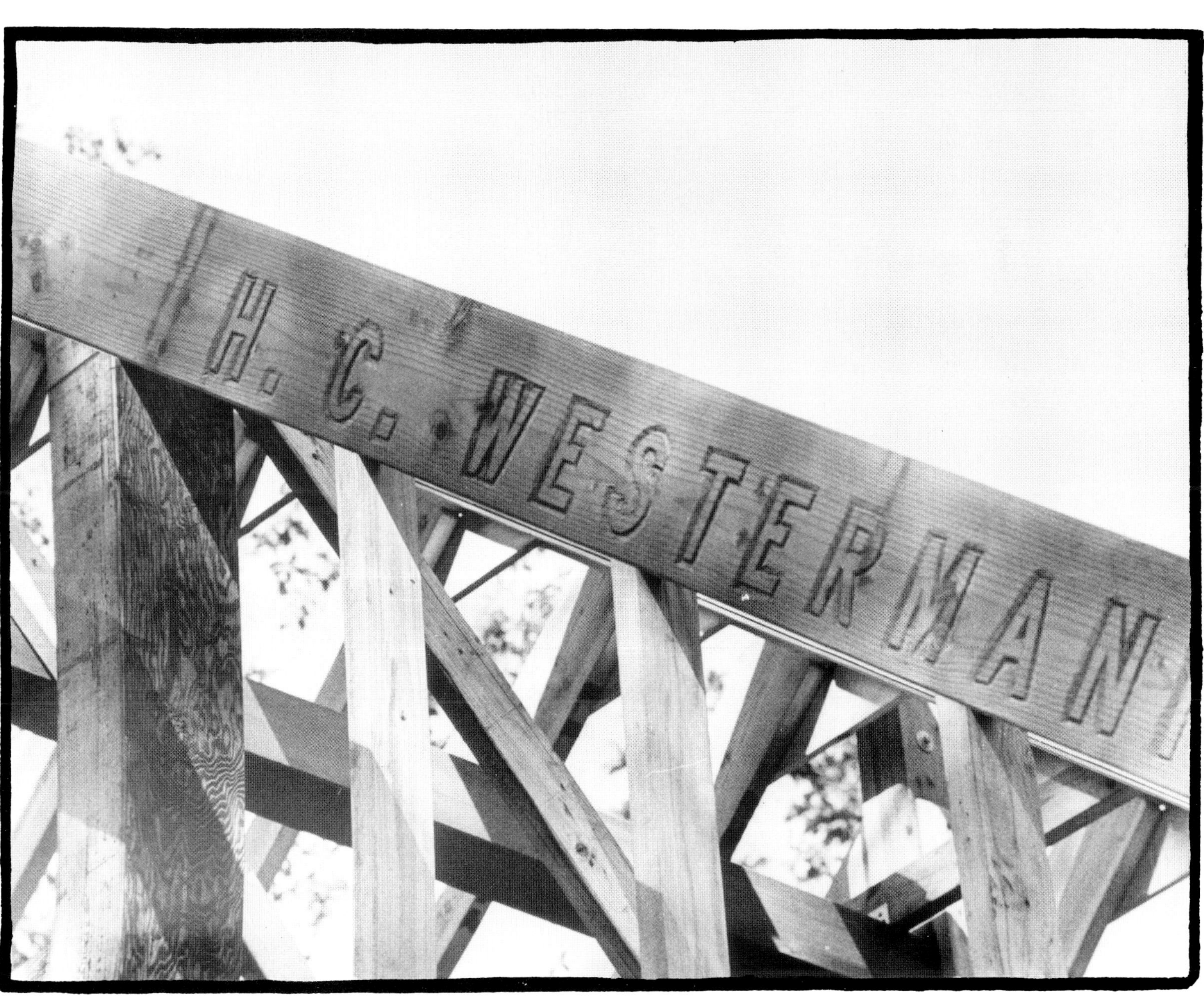

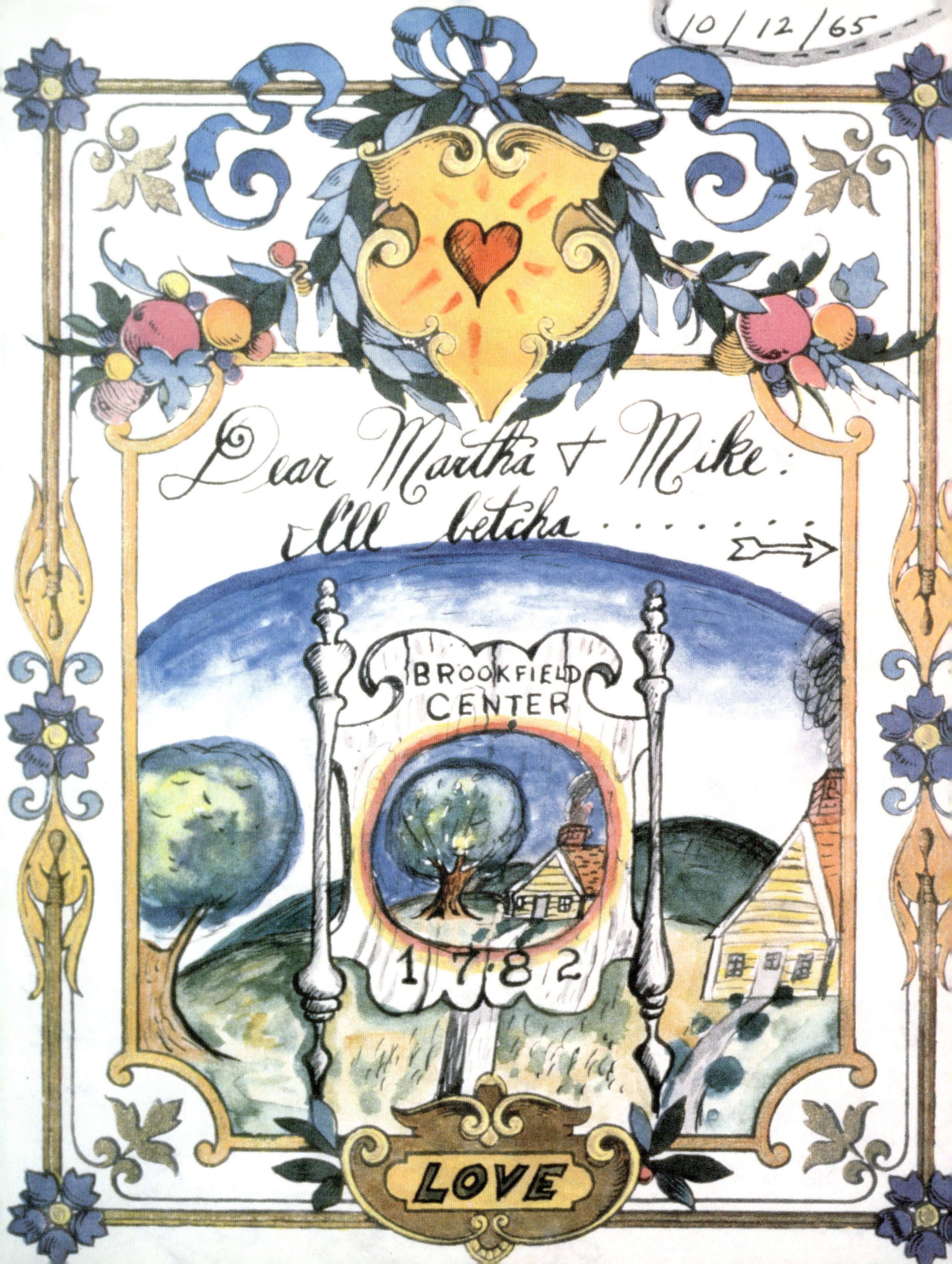
10/12/65
Dear Martha & Mike:
I'll betcha
BROOKFIELD CENTER
1782
LOVE

from a letter to Bruce + Doris Oxford December 27, 1967

Well ole Joanny + I are fine + we keep out of the pool hall. I built her a chimney this summer (Aug 8th - Nov 8th) + it's shaped liked a whiskey bottle + has five concrete mushrooms on top. That's too big a job for one man + the labor reminded me of you guys when you were bustin' your asses at 222. I worked night + day too on the "THING". She now has a great huge room of her own with an 18′ ceiling inside (25′ × 36′) + it's like a cathedral. I didn't build the room only the chimney. She's doing all the interior work + painting inside + out.

from a letter to Herk and Diana van Tongeren November 4, 1971

I don't know whether I mentioned it but I'm building my shop, my wife + I that is, + I'm putting the firring strips up on the rafters now for the shingles. The main structural joints are all mortised + tenoned (Douglas fir, 6 × 8, with double red wood sill). It takes a lot of time you know. + I ended up bolting the studs to the joists (floor + ceiling) + have used a thousand bolts. Wood shingles + all the structural pieces were treated with woodlife or creosote. I gotta get my ass going some up there, to get it covered over. I'll make it.

from a letter to Martha and Mike Renner September 3, 1981

We have been working seven days a week on the house, night + day for months + expect to move in in Oct. sometime .... Of course with this house the most important aspect, of course, is what you don't see, in a sense. By that I mean the basic framework, or structure, as you wish. It was done right. Every stud + every rafter + header, etc. The whole thing has been done right. Oh incidentally we are screwing the flooring down with 2½″ #12 or #14 flat head brass screws, flush with the surface. They look swell + really do the job.

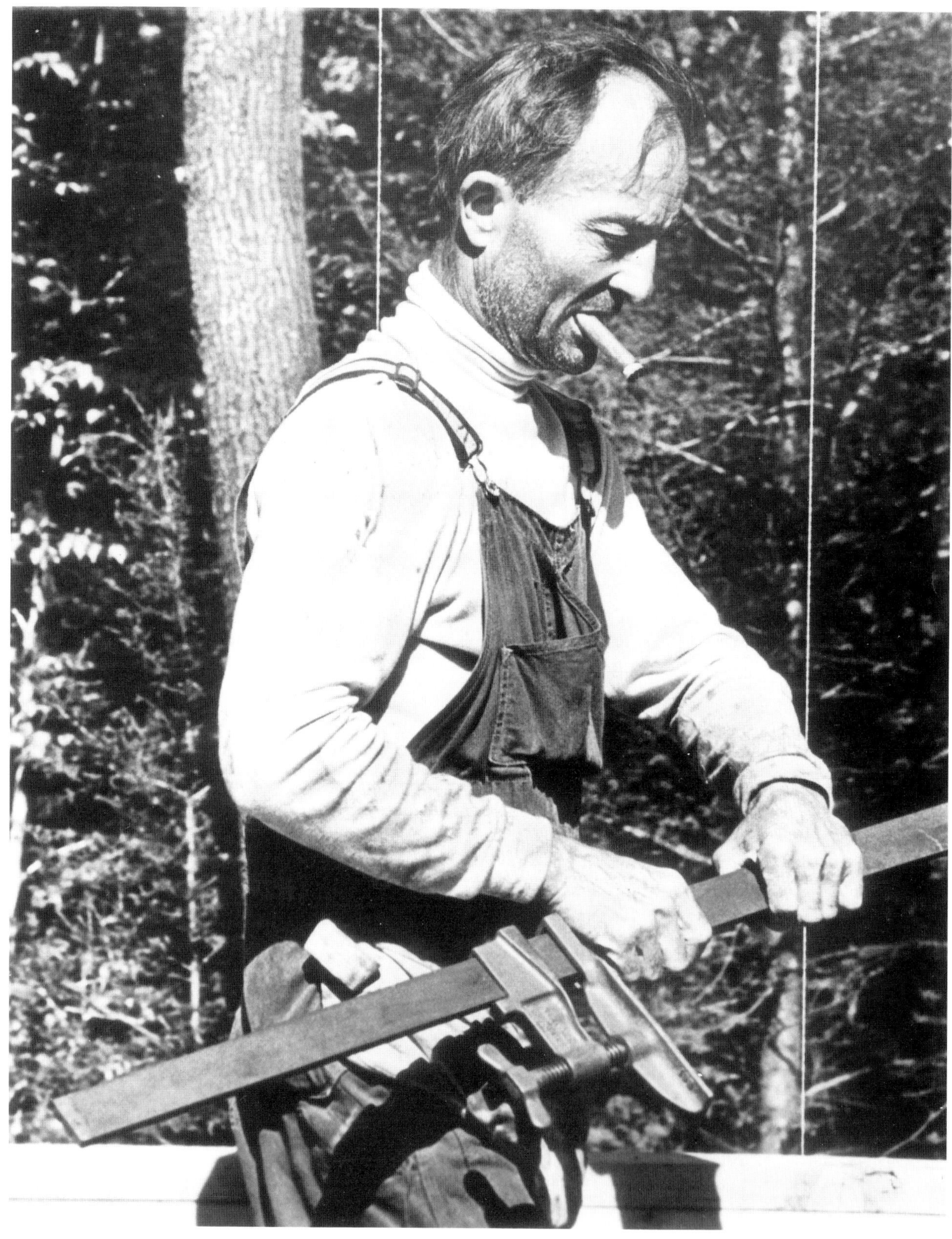

Westermann working on the house in Brookfield Center, 1971

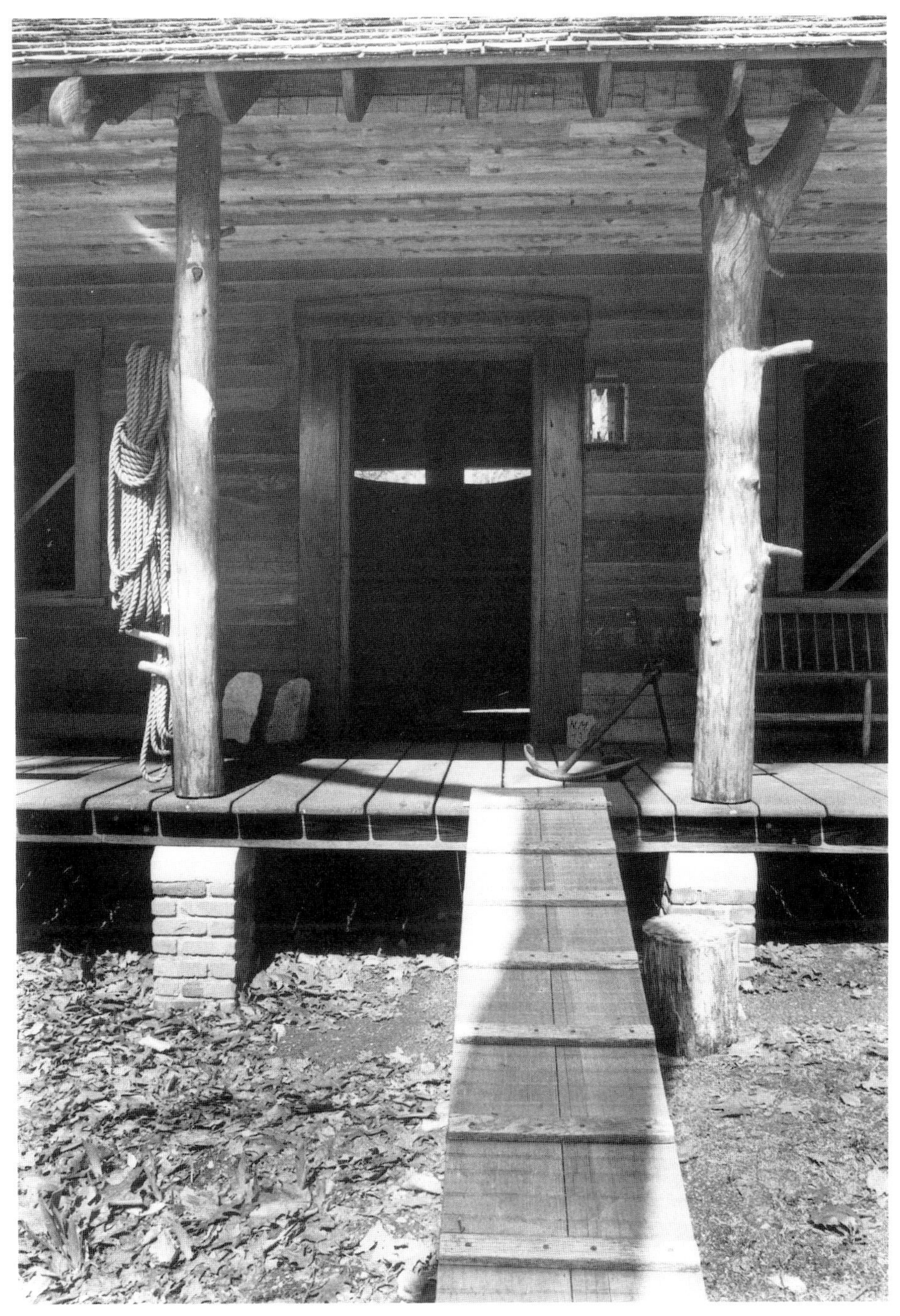

Entrance to the house in Brookfield Center

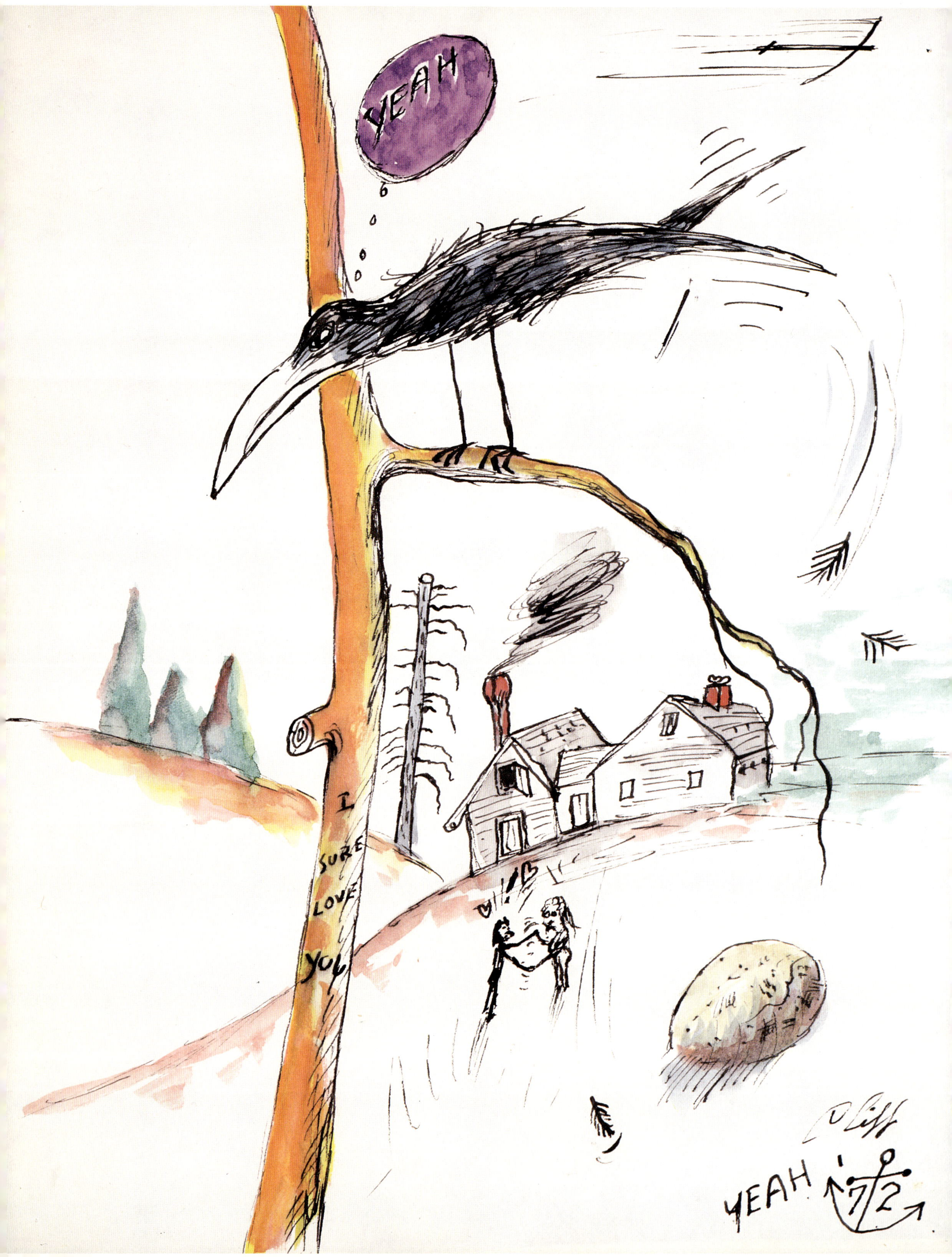
YEAH
I
SURE
LOVE
YOU
YEAH

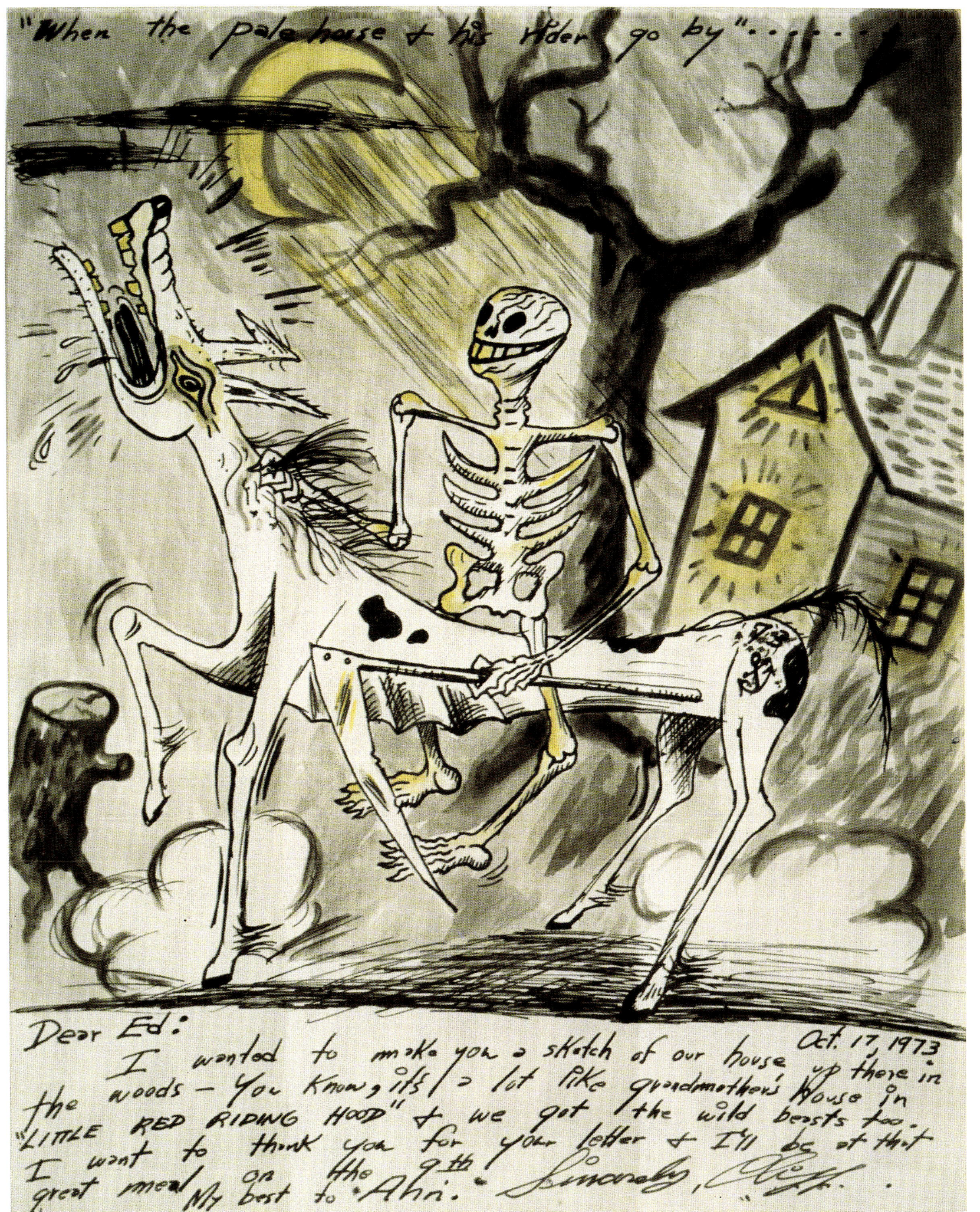

"When the pale horse & his rider go by"......
Dear Ed:
Oct. 17, 1973
I wanted to make you a sketch of our house up there in the woods — You know, it's a lot like grandmother's House in "LITTLE RED RIDING HOOD" & we got the wild beasts too.
I want to thank you for your letter & I'll be at that great meal on the 9th!
My best to "Ahn."
Sincerely, Cliff.

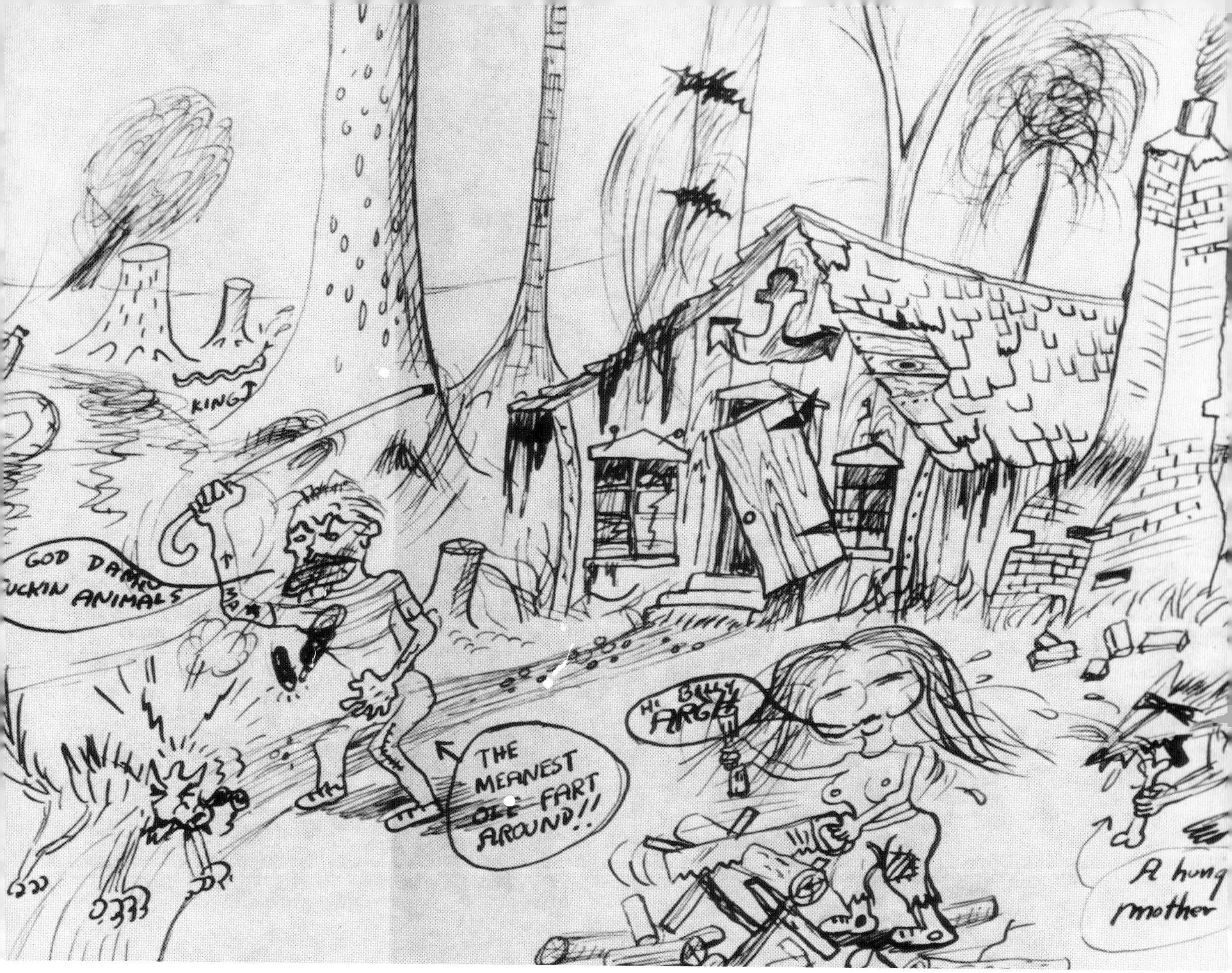

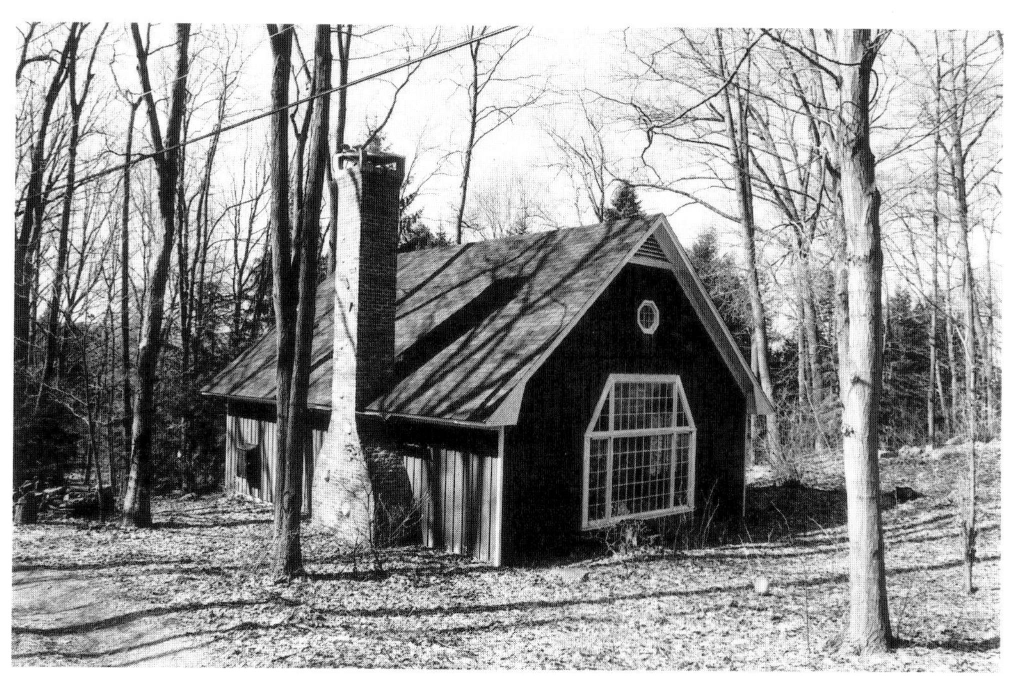

Joanna's studio with chimney built by Westermann

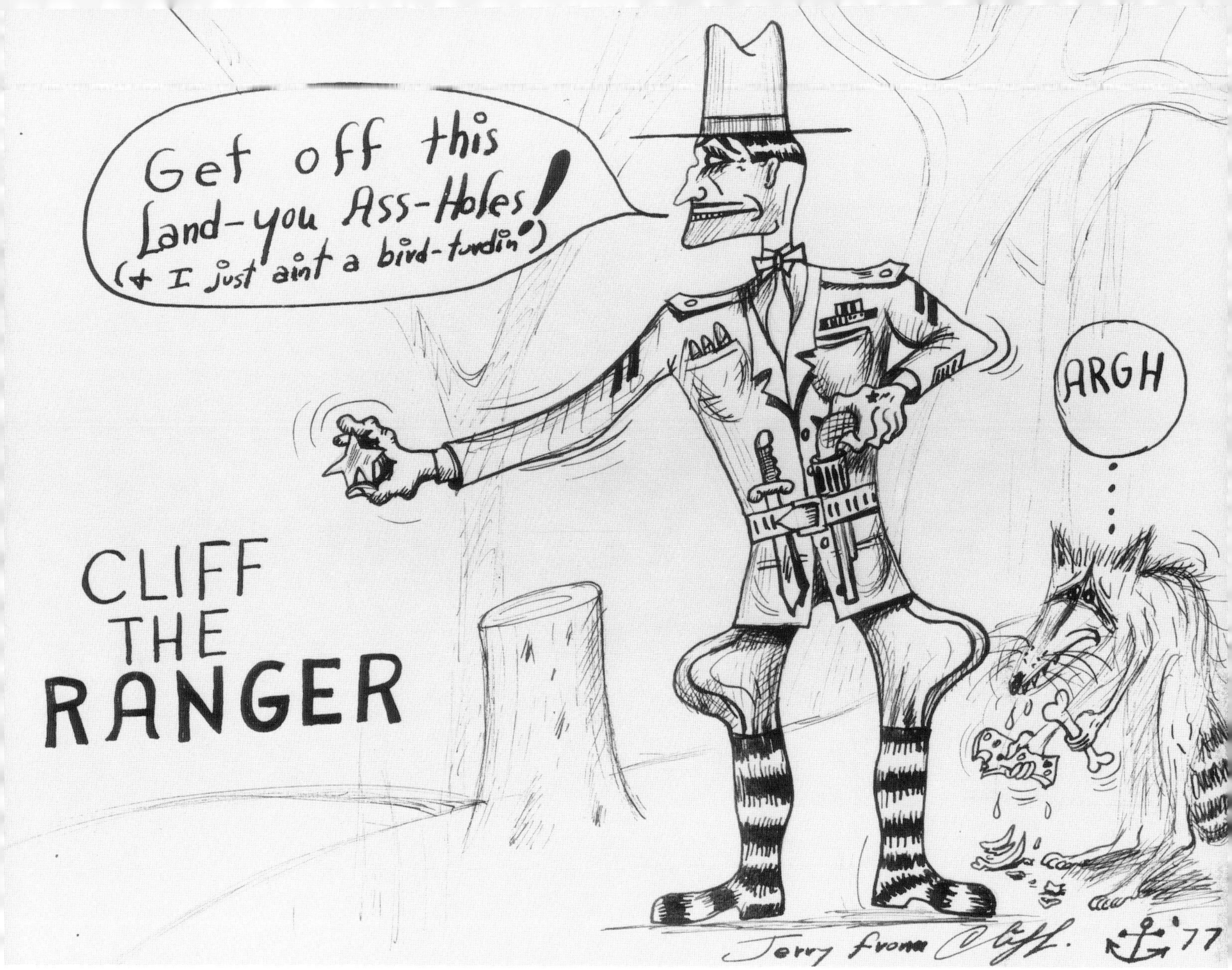

Get off this
Land-you Ass-Holes!
(+ I just aint a bird-turdin'!)

ARGH

CLIFF
THE
RANGER

Jerry from Cliff. '77

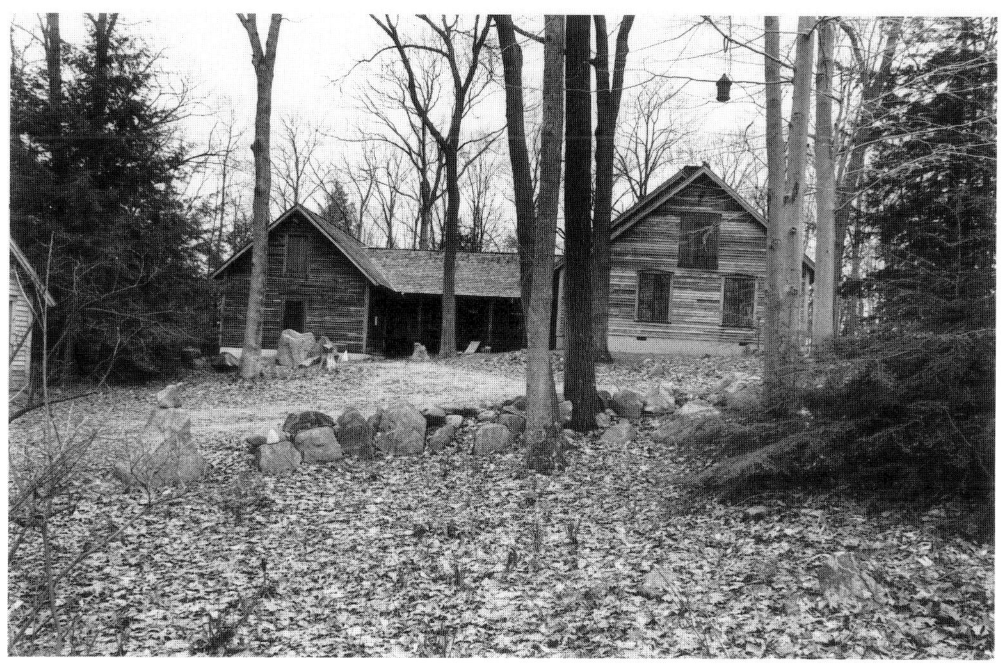

Westermann's studio and house in Brookfield Center

June 21, 1981

Dear Gene:

The other night I was sitting up there on my swing — it was a full moon + perfectly still. I suddenly could swear I heard you four people laughing + thumping around + working like hell in the house + that plaster machine was running. You know, all those great plastering noises. It was pretty weird — an interesting + exciting experience. Well you four great ones have been gone a little over a week now + we sure miss you people — your beautiful well organized work schedule, your spirits of good cheer + your great skills. All of you. We miss your fine attitudes towards your work + your friendliness towards us. Gene, it was the chance of a lifetime to see something really beautiful being done, on the spot. Your job is a masterpiece + each day we come to realize that more. I'm convinced you are the only four men, in the whole fucking world, that could have done such a perfect beautiful job. Joanny has the plastic all off now + has been working on the outlet boxes + the floors + I have been helping her a little too. The first thing I do in the morning when I go up there early — is to stroll through the whole house just admiring the great job, much to my enjoyment. Well, we miss you people considerably but the job is done. I hope all of you took on a good new job. We'll never forget you fine people. You are rare ones. This is Bus's shirt + we all took a crack at trying to remove the plaster. We're still battling those mother-fucking bugs + they ended up defoliating everything including the top of my head; but as you said Gene: their shit is great fertilizer. (That's not much consolation). The best to you all. I hope Primo's wife is steadily growing stronger + tell Billy I love that electrical box he gave me + have been using it steadily. Keep your hawk clean Gene + all my best.

Cliff

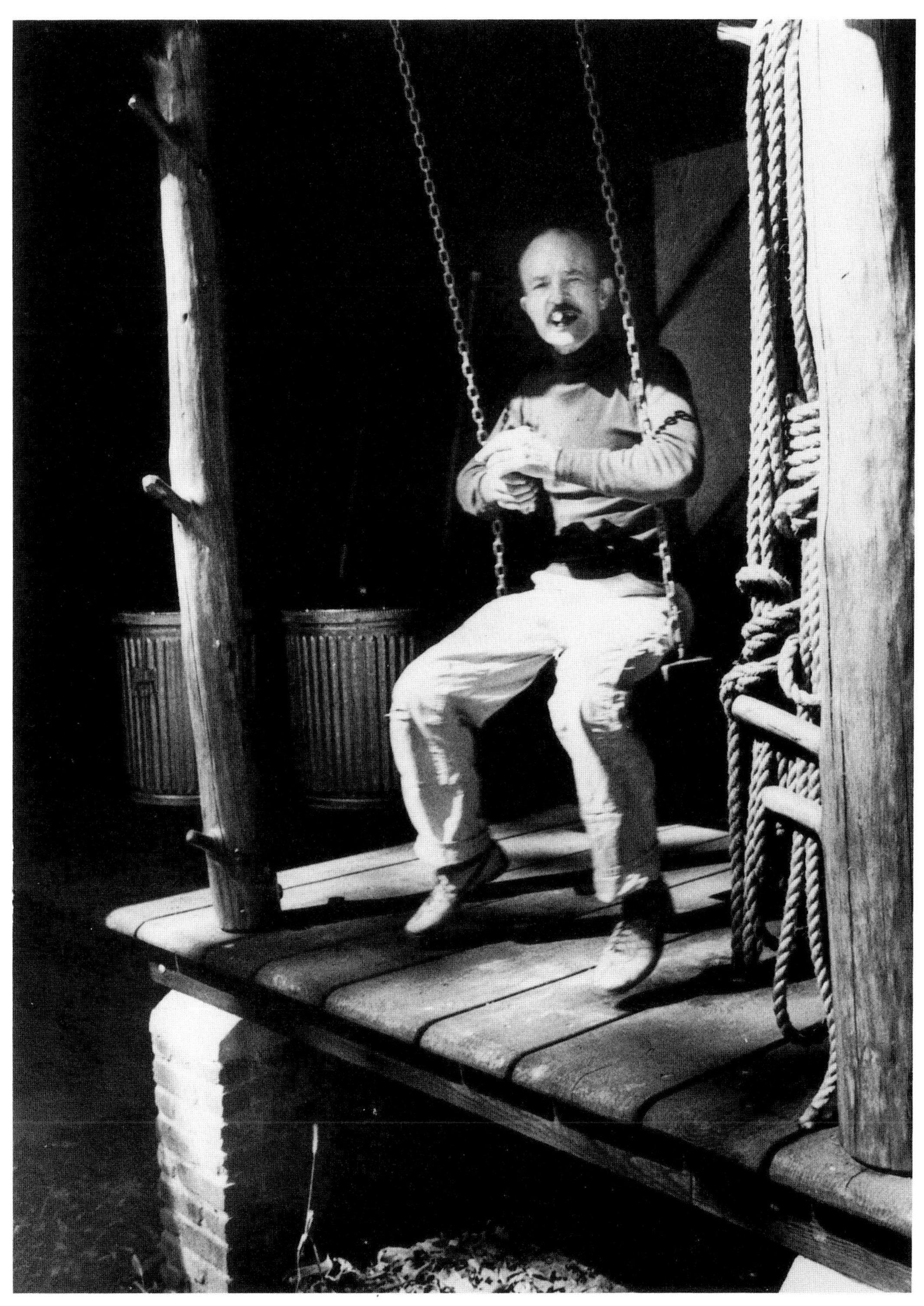

Westermann on the front porch of his house, summer 1981

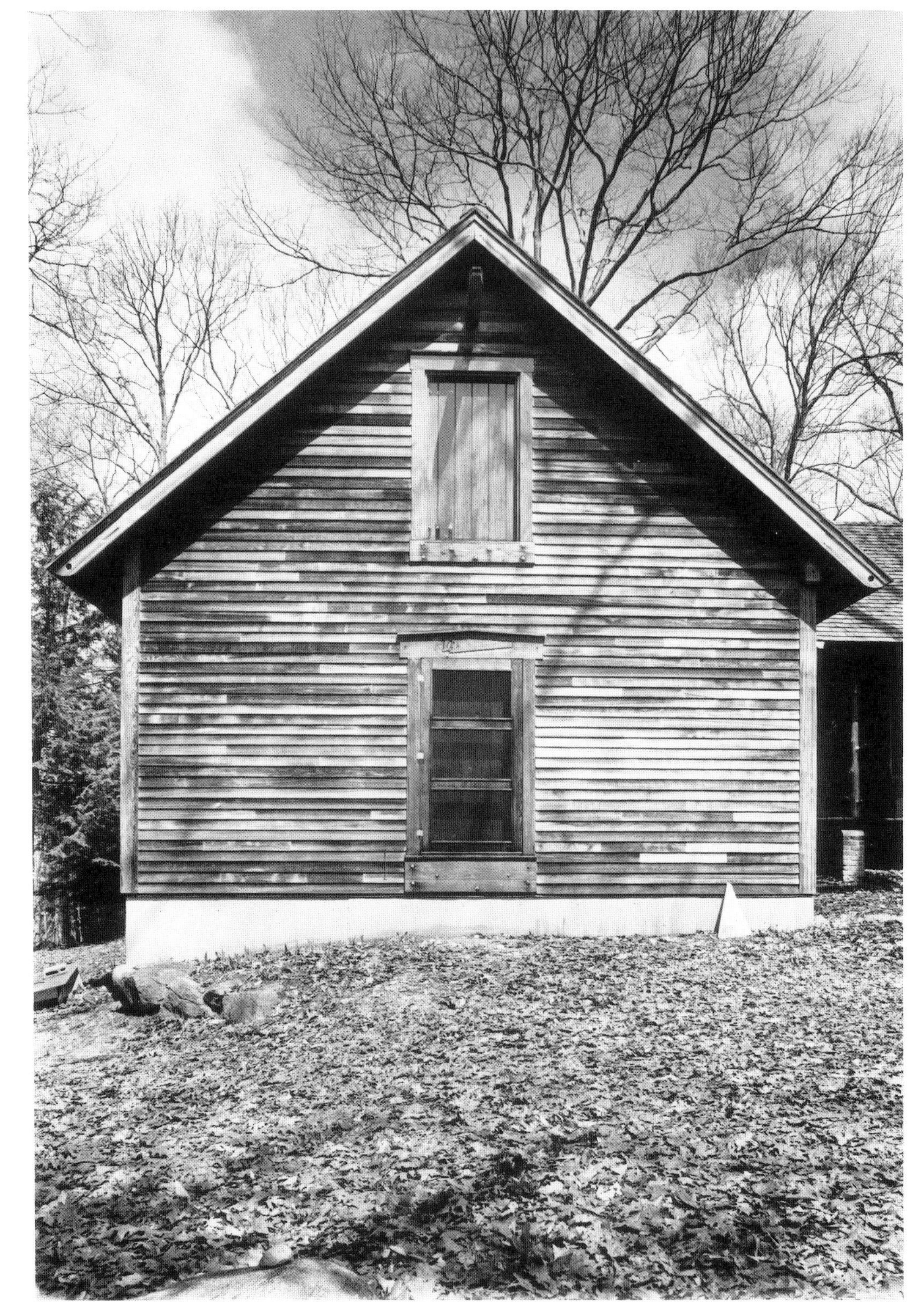

Westermann's studio in Brookfield Center

October 30, 1981

Dear Ruth:

I imagine you would recognize that wire lath on the piece. I have an idea that Mr. Grenzbach used that in your house, in Cheriot Knolls, before it was plastered? Or did he use wood lath? I can't quite remember. Anyway we had wire lath used in our house in every room + then of course a 3 course plaster job (scratch coat, brown coat, + then the white coat). They did a beautiful job in the guest room, living room, + master bedroom. We had them make a real nice cornice, which, of course was plaster, + that is an interesting technique. They do it with a tin cross-section of the finish cornice + pull it across through the wet plaster of paris right in front of him (the plaster of paris being placed by another workmen. The inside + outside corners are especially difficult, it turned out just exquisite + Gene, the boss, told me that ours was the first complete house with plaster walls ¾″ thick + the cornice that they had done in 35 years. Gene + his crew got pretty excited with the job. The way they have managed to keep going all these years, as plasterers, is mainly restoration work or repairs of sections, etc. I'm pretty sure we will finally be able to move in in Nov. My buddy came up from N.Y. (he is a sculptor + carpenter) + stayed here for 8 weeks. We put the oak floor down, some of the planks were 17″ wide — they averaged about 13″. We bought that oak 12 years ago + it is perfectly seasoned. We did a swell job of it + Joanny has been putting the finish on it (Watco + wax) + it's beautiful. We were lucky + got a fantastic cabinet maker to do the cabinets in the kitchen + pantry. Joanny's delight. The tile in the bathroom is beautiful. It's Italian + French. The kitchen floor is French terracotta tile + it's beautiful too. It came from an area in Southern France where they have been making this type of tile for 300 years + a limited amount because they are hand made. They sift the dry clay 3 times to remove the impurities before they start to make the tiles + then it is high fired. That tile is very elegant. All of the plumbing is copper or bronze + the fixtures are 1st class. There are <u>no</u> mickey-mouse materials in the house. My really hard jobs are done + I can coast now. Oh I have inside doors to make + trim work inside, but I can do these things at my leisure. I think it turned out beautiful far beyond our expectations, I think because we never compromised on materials + details such as hinges, all brass, etc. Down to the last detail. Eventually we'll send you some photos of the place. You know it's been 12 years now since we started this house — Ruth + structurally I guess it's about the strongest house in Conn., including some of the old Colonial gems. We think of you a lot Ruth + I hope you had a nice summer.

Love,
Cliff

Death Ships

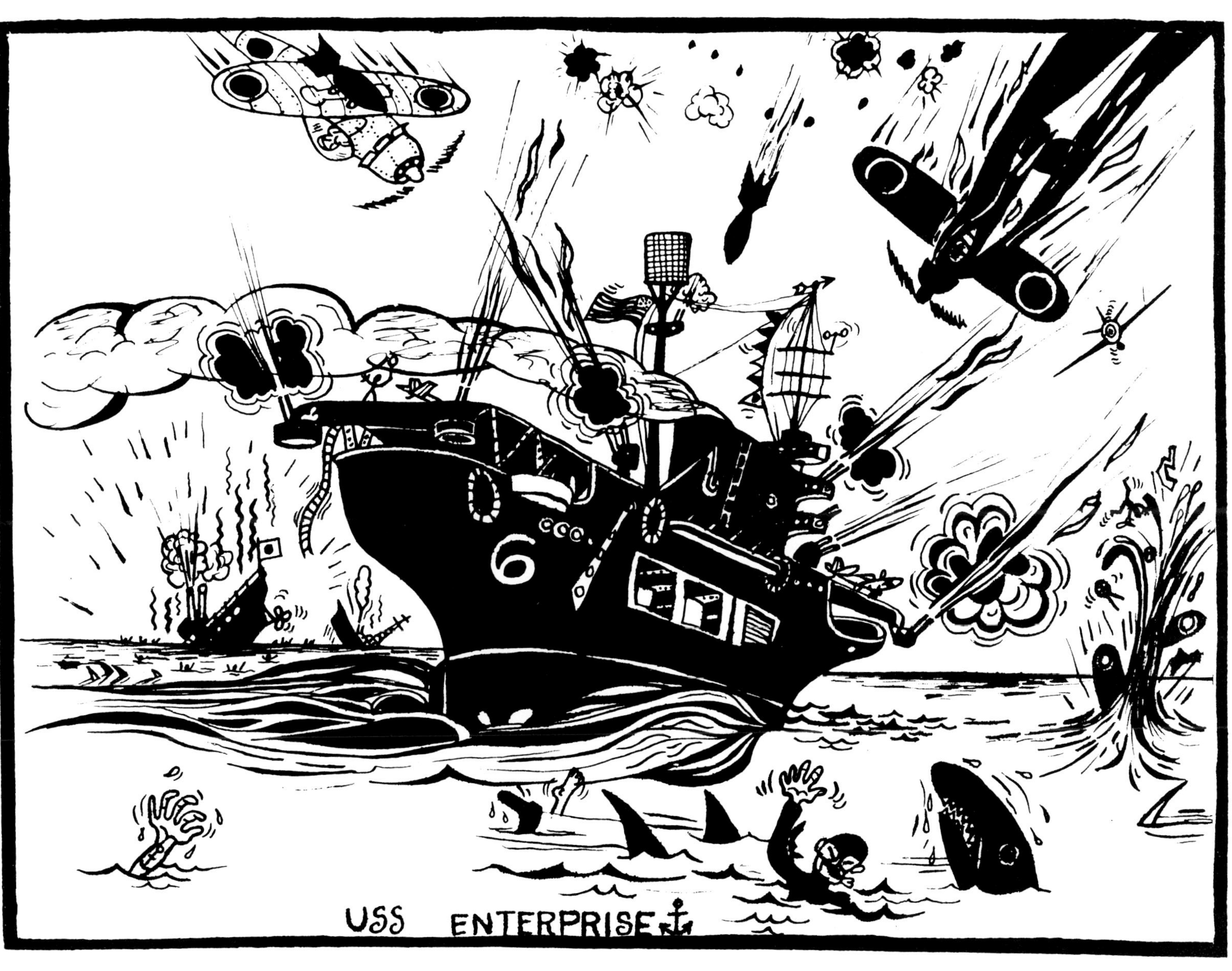

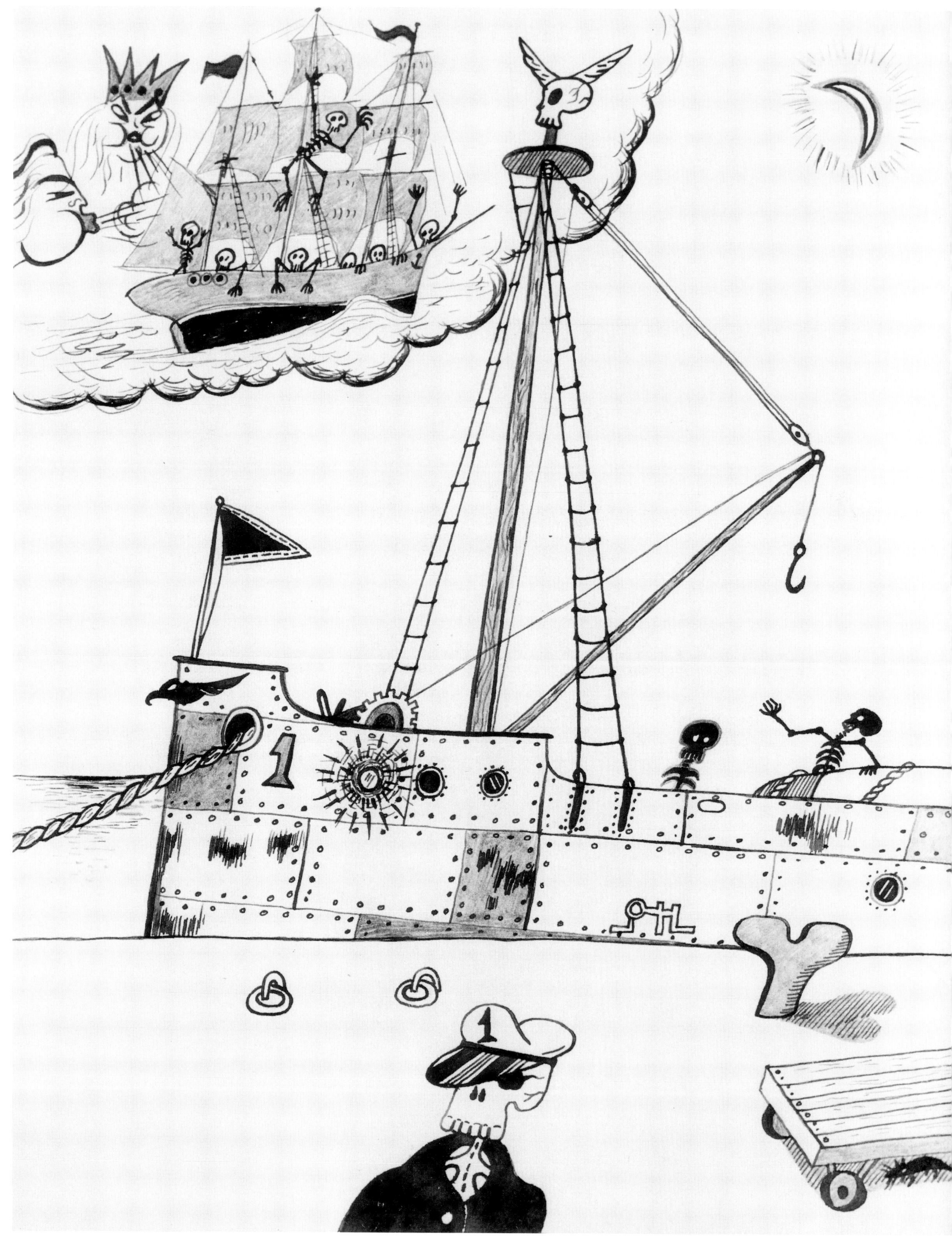

April 14, 1971

Dear Herk:

Thanks for your nice letter + that's swell you got that teaching job. I want you to know I sure enjoy the beautiful anchor you sent me + I'll take good care of it. I got a little painting here that I did in about 1935 (when I was a kid) of a ship, the "Great Eastern", I believe. I used to try + draw them + make ship models + none of them were any good, very frustrating, but I love to do it anyhow. I lived in L.A. + the harbor there was San Pedro about 25 miles away. I used to spend days down there just looking around + you wouldn't believe it but I used to see old wooden sailing vessels come in + their cargo was lumber from Oregon + Washington + Alaska. They were coastal vessels + then some of them were wooden steamships. At that time they had no anchor fences + you could walk all over there + nobody would bother you. This was in the 30's of course. Gee how I used to love to watch them unload that great lumber + timbers. It was the "real McCoy" — Now it's bullshit + they got those lousy fences everplace. You know. + then I went North when I was a kid + worked in the logging camps + sawmills. Very mysterious. I guess I always loved ships + they come natural + once I was aboard a carrier for over a year without stepping foot off it. This was once during WW II. But that never bothered me. I like the sea + feel at home there. But then I have seen "Death Ships", many of them + I can't get them out of my lousy system. You know how it is! Well I still make those ships + I am a 48 year old fart. + they still aren't very good, but now I don't give a damn + they satisfy some kind of need there — But they are all death ships now. Forgive me kid.

Good luck!!

Sincerely,
H.C. Westermann

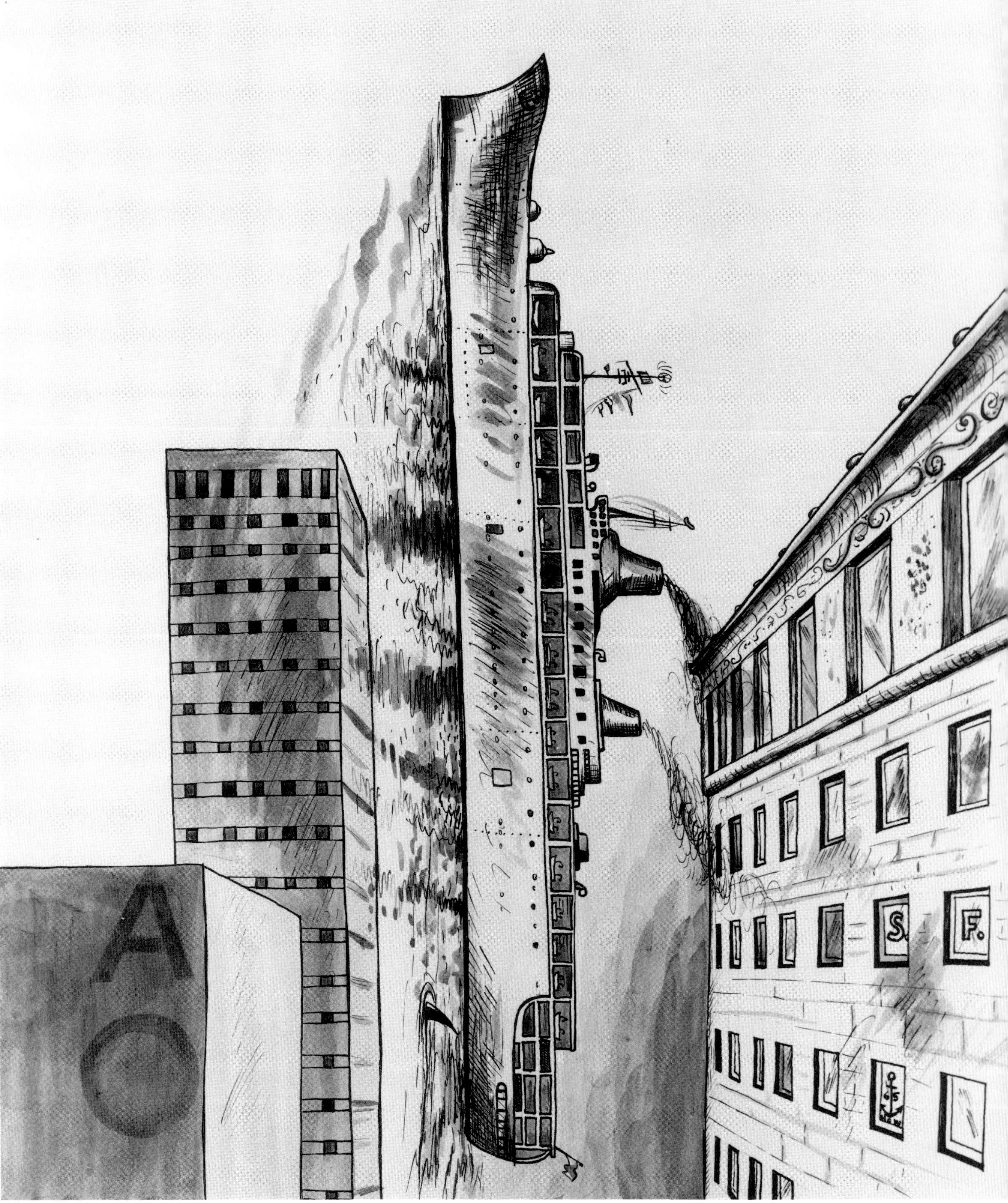
A
O
S
F.

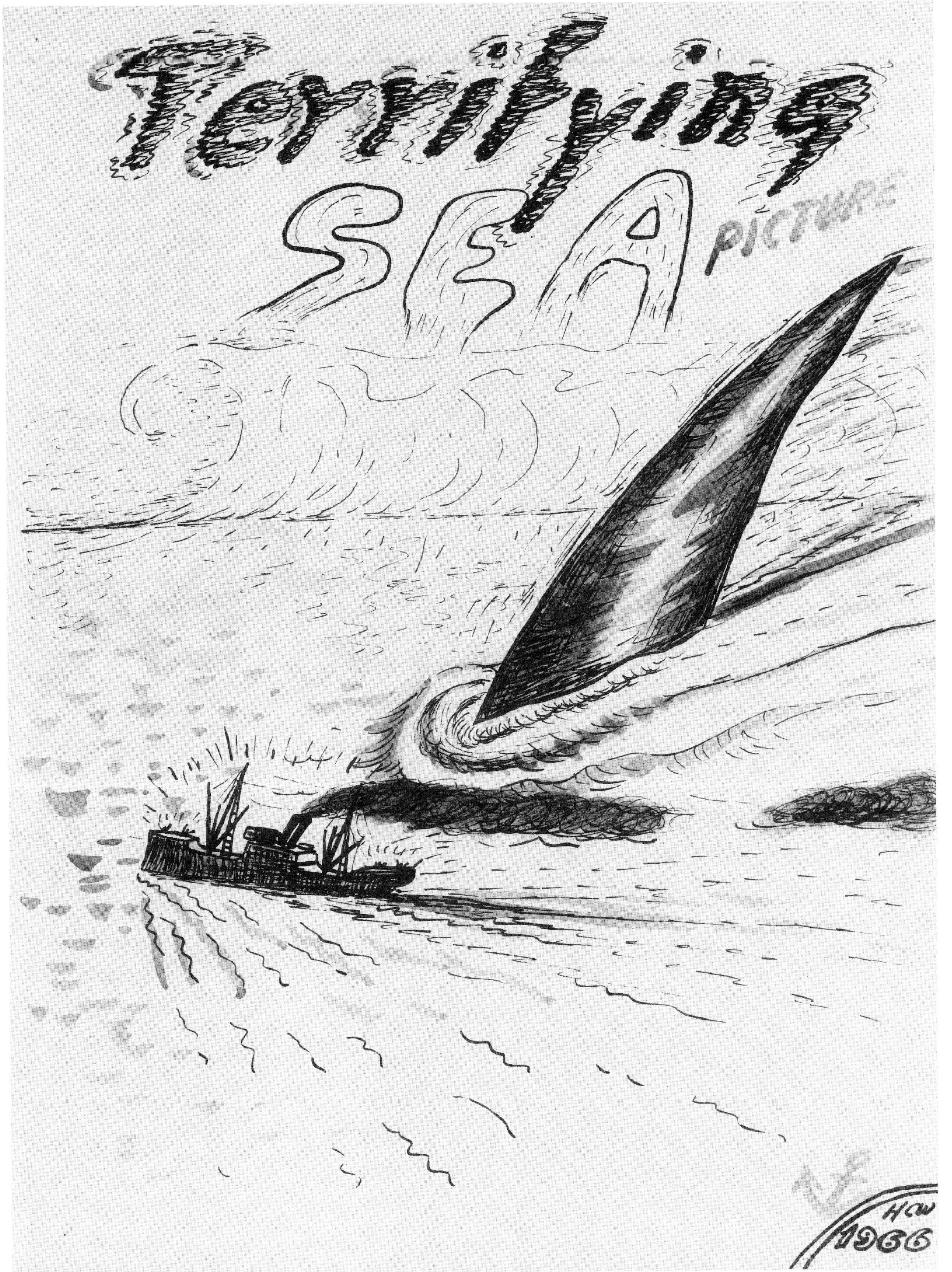

Terrifying
SEA
PICTURE
HCW
1966

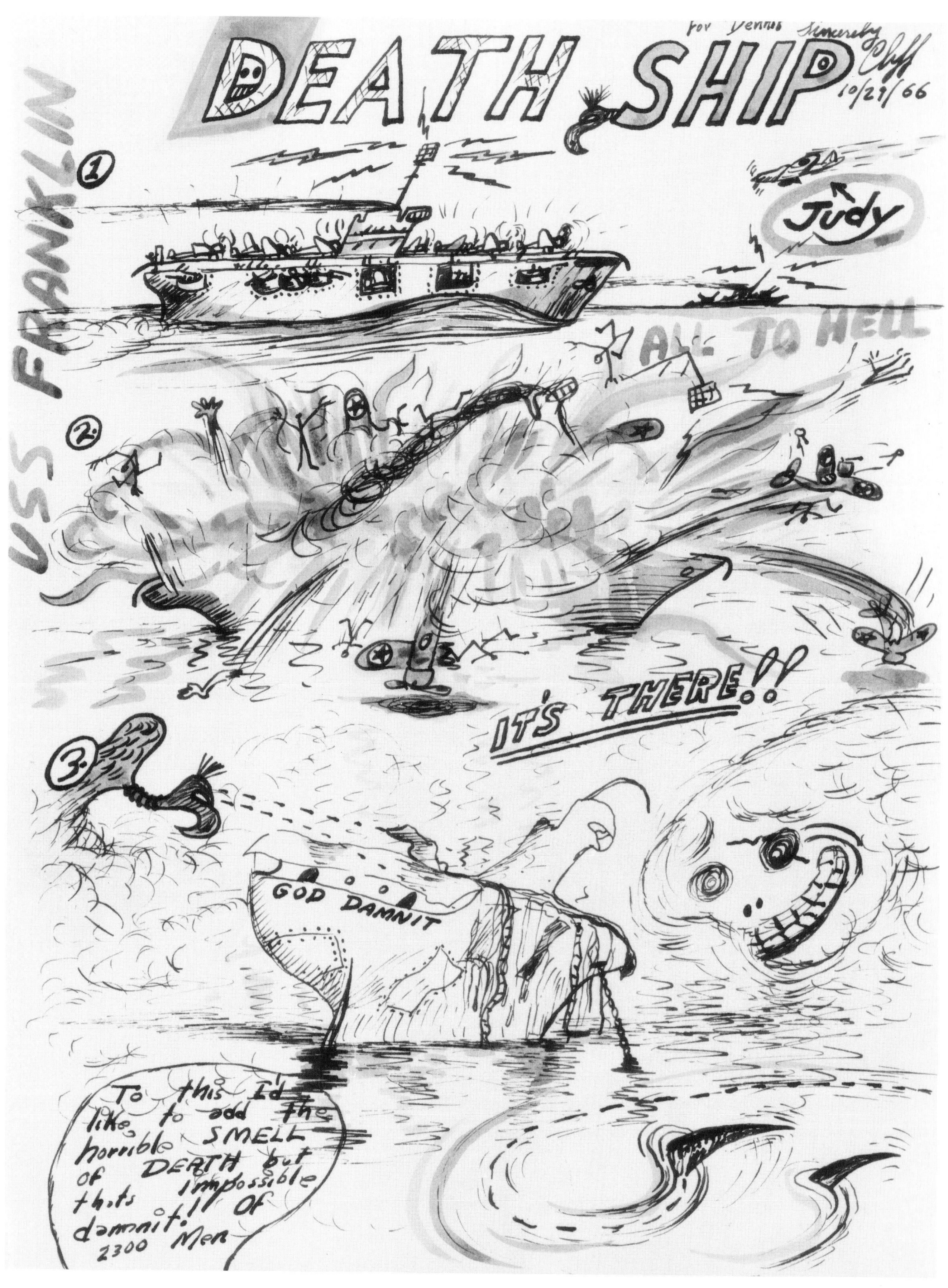
for Dennis Sincerely Cliff 10/29/66
DEATH SHIP
USS FRANKLIN
1
Judy
ALL TO HELL
2
IT'S THERE!!
3
GOD DAMNIT
To this I'd like to add the horrible SMELL of DEATH but thats impossible damnit! !! Of 2300 Men

Dear Norma: I want to thank you for the invitation - I couldn't make it. I haven't read the Odyssey yet but I will - Anyway here's a make believe picture of it ? "In Hoc Signo Vinces" - which means in Greek "Together we stand, united we FALL?" ©

11/8/66

ODYSSEY

This is a sort of form letter & elevated just one small step above "junk mail."

EVERY YEAR (15) SHIPS OF OVER 500 TONS VANISH FROM THE FACE OF THE EARTH WITHOUT A TRACE & NO SURVIVORS. TRUE!

say hello to Bill.

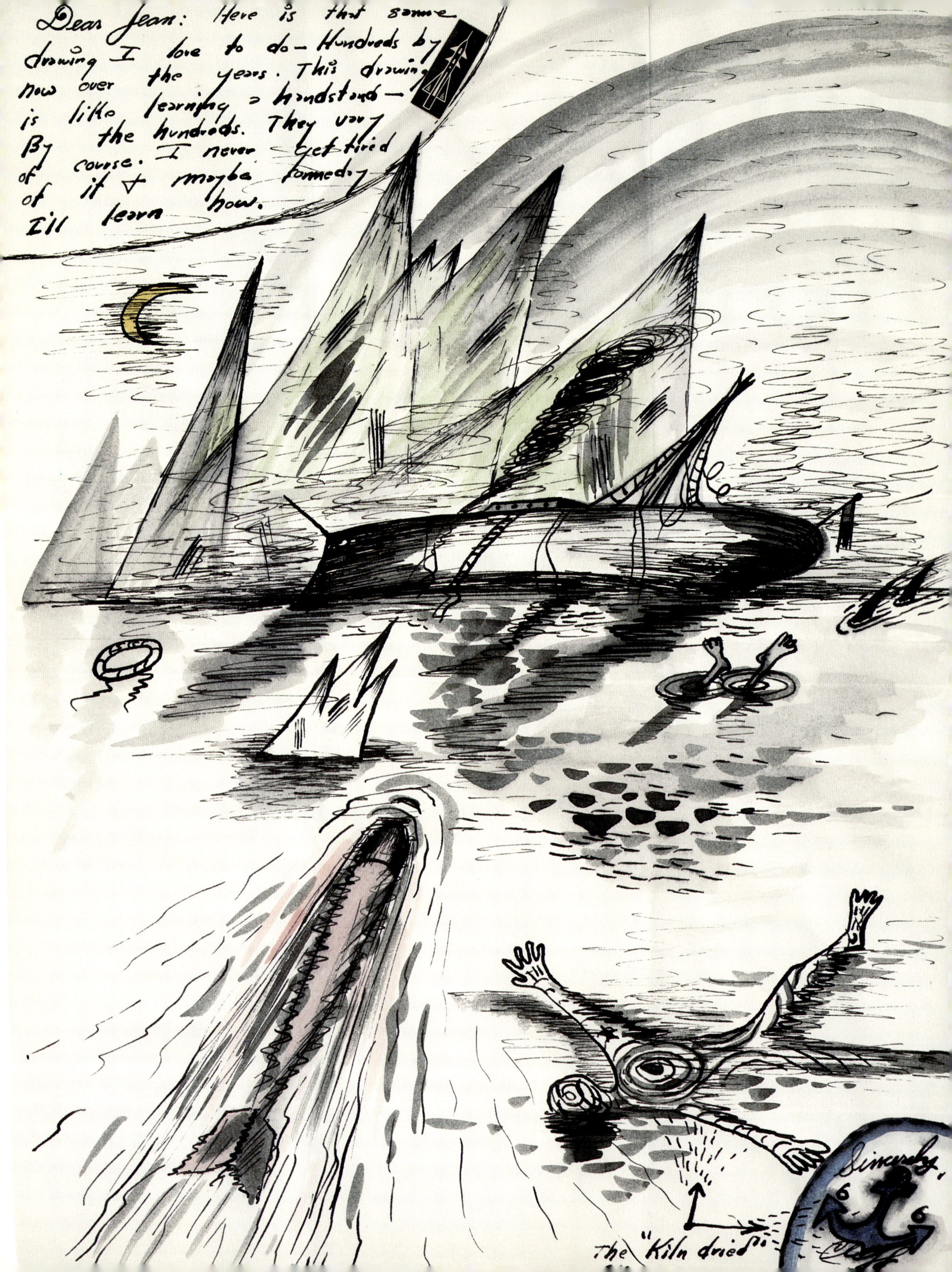
Dear Jean: Here is that same
drawing I love to do — Hundreds by
now over the years. This drawing
is like learning a handstand —
By the hundreds. They vary
of course. I never get tired
of it + maybe someday
I'll learn how.
the "Kiln dried"
Sincerely,

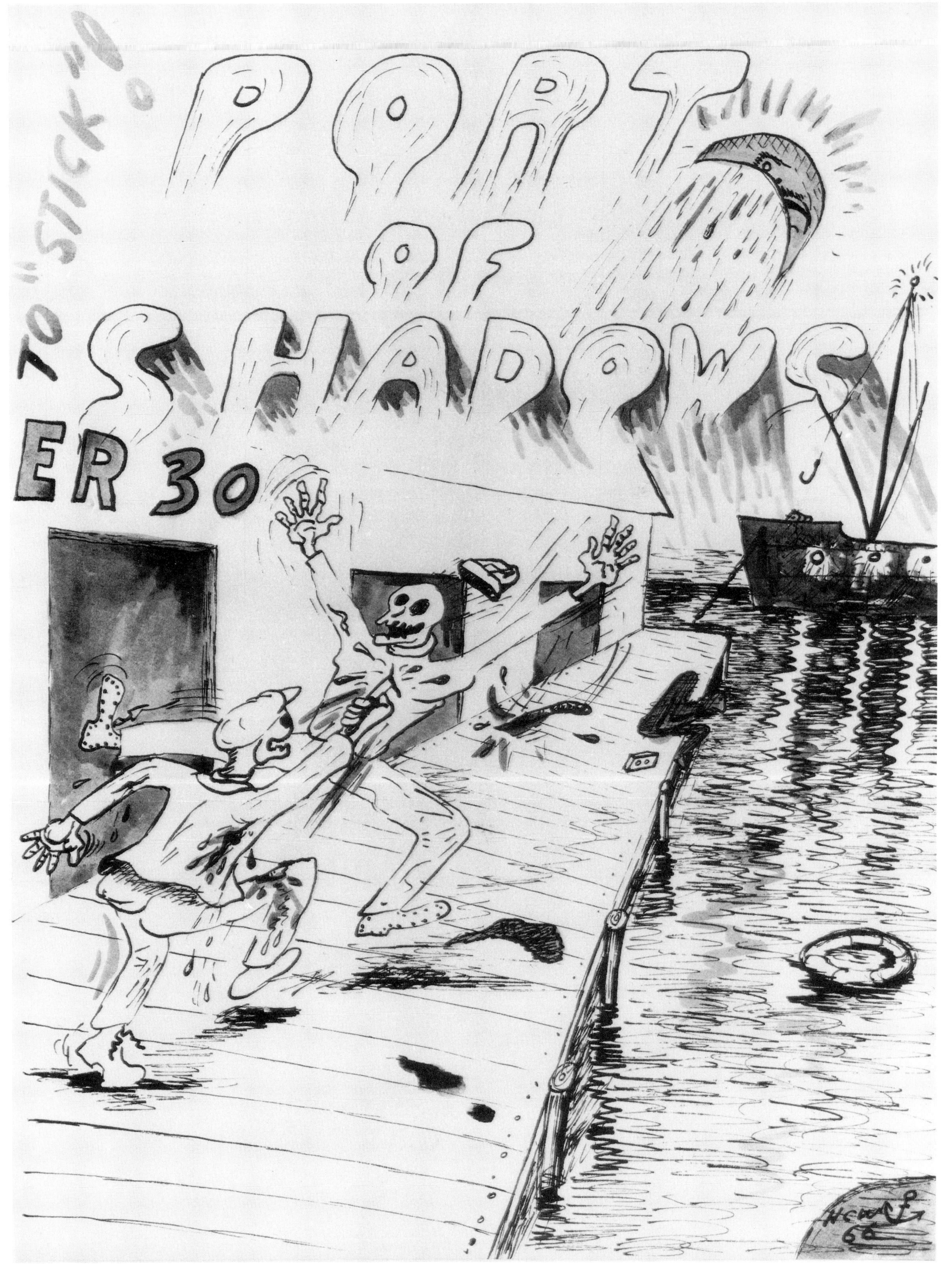
TO "STICK" O'
PORT OF SHADOWS
ER 30
HCW 66

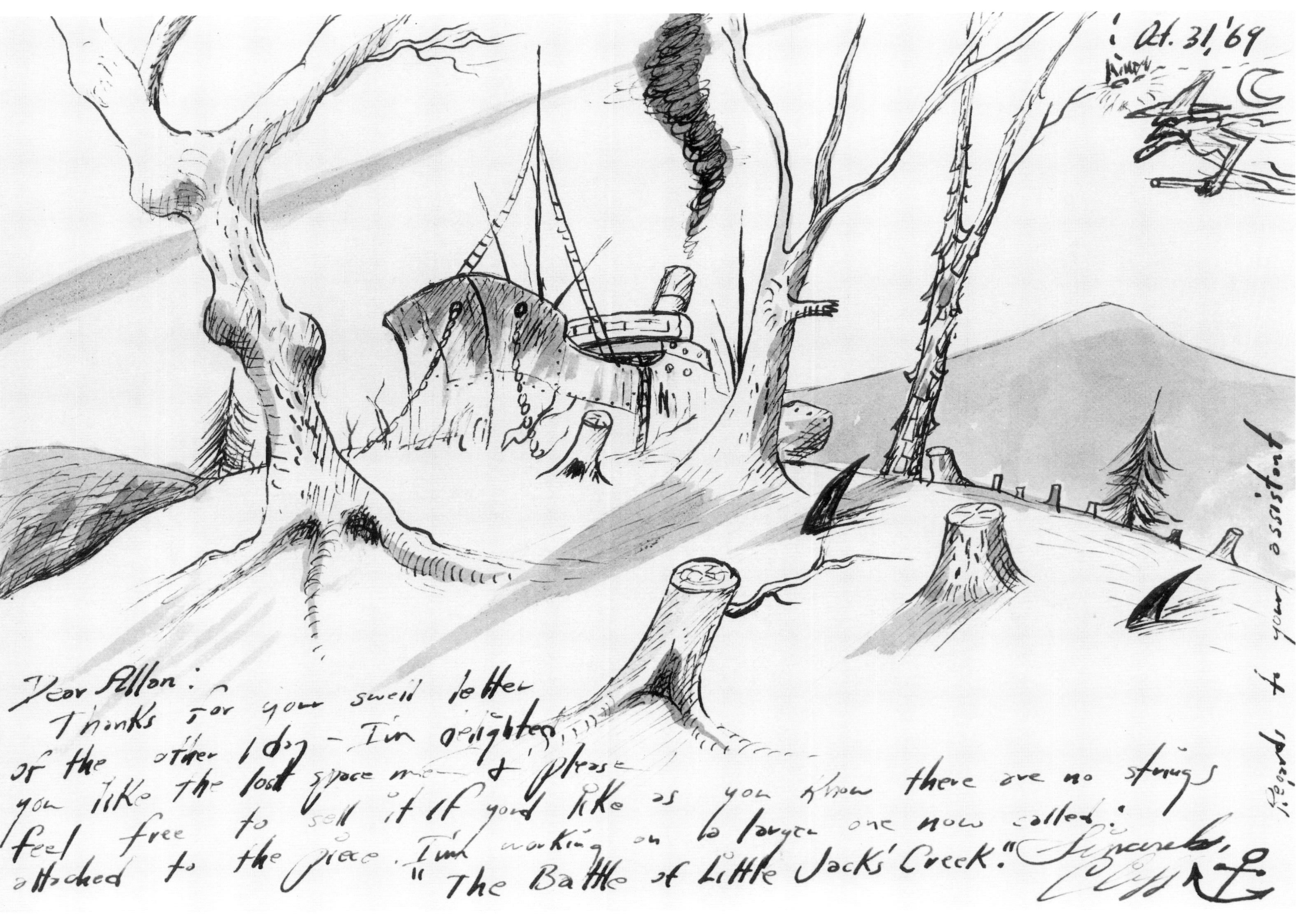
Oct. 31, '69
Dear Allan:
Thanks for your swell letter
of the other day - I'm delighted
you like the lost space men & please
feel free to sell it if you'd like as you know there are no strings
attached to the piece. I'm working on a larger one now called:
"The Battle of Little Jacks' Creek."
Sincerely,
Cliff
Regards to your assistant

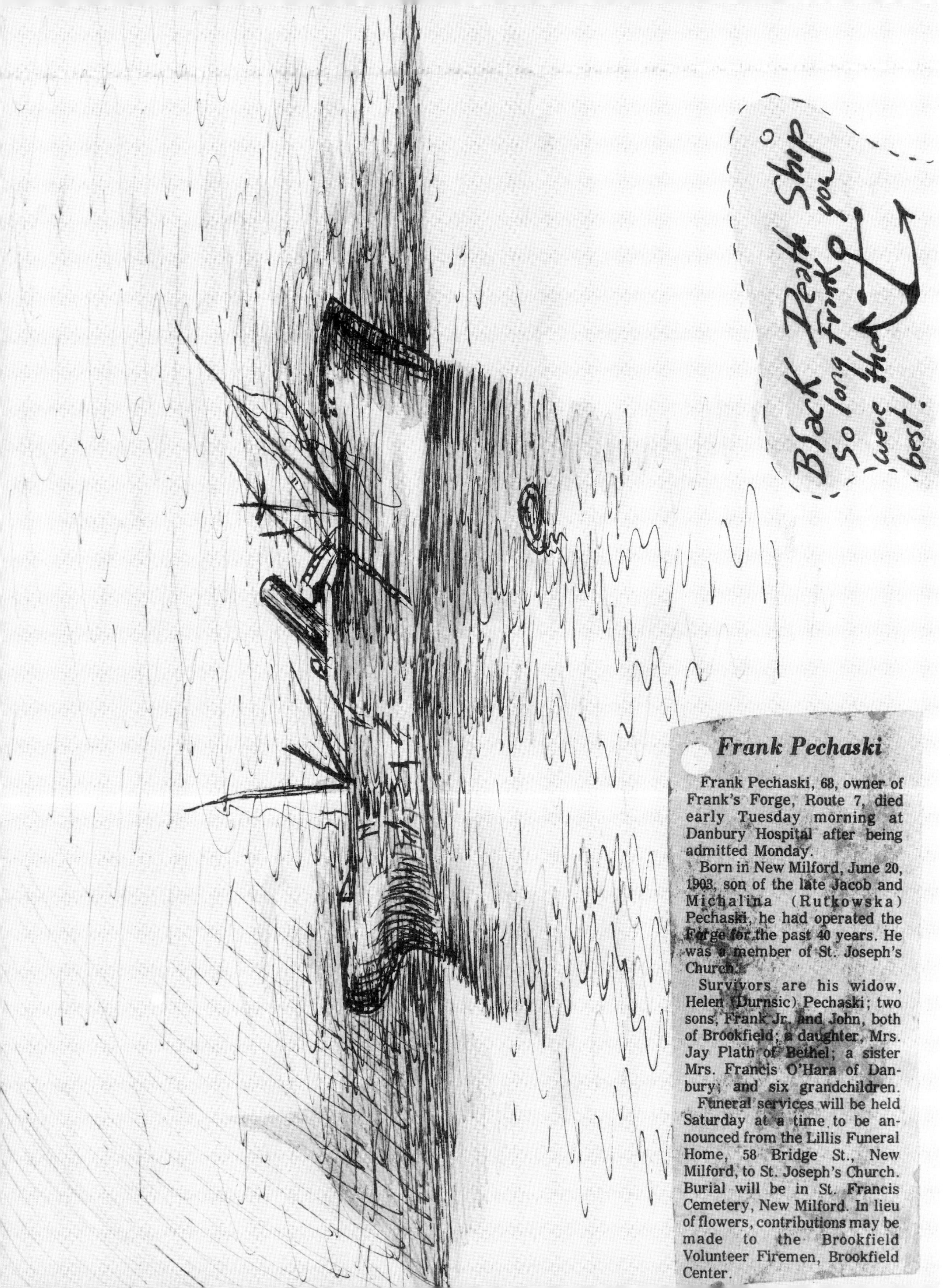

Frank Pechaski

Frank Pechaski, 68, owner of Frank's Forge, Route 7, died early Tuesday morning at Danbury Hospital after being admitted Monday.

Born in New Milford, June 20, 1903, son of the late Jacob and Michalina (Rutkowska) Pechaski, he had operated the Forge for the past 40 years. He was a member of St. Joseph's Church.

Survivors are his widow, Helen (Durnsic) Pechaski; two sons, Frank Jr. and John, both of Brookfield; a daughter, Mrs. Jay Plath of Bethel; a sister Mrs. Francis O'Hara of Danbury; and six grandchildren.

Funeral services will be held Saturday at a time to be announced from the Lillis Funeral Home, 58 Bridge St., New Milford, to St. Joseph's Church. Burial will be in St. Francis Cemetery, New Milford. In lieu of flowers, contributions may be made to the Brookfield Volunteer Firemen, Brookfield Center.

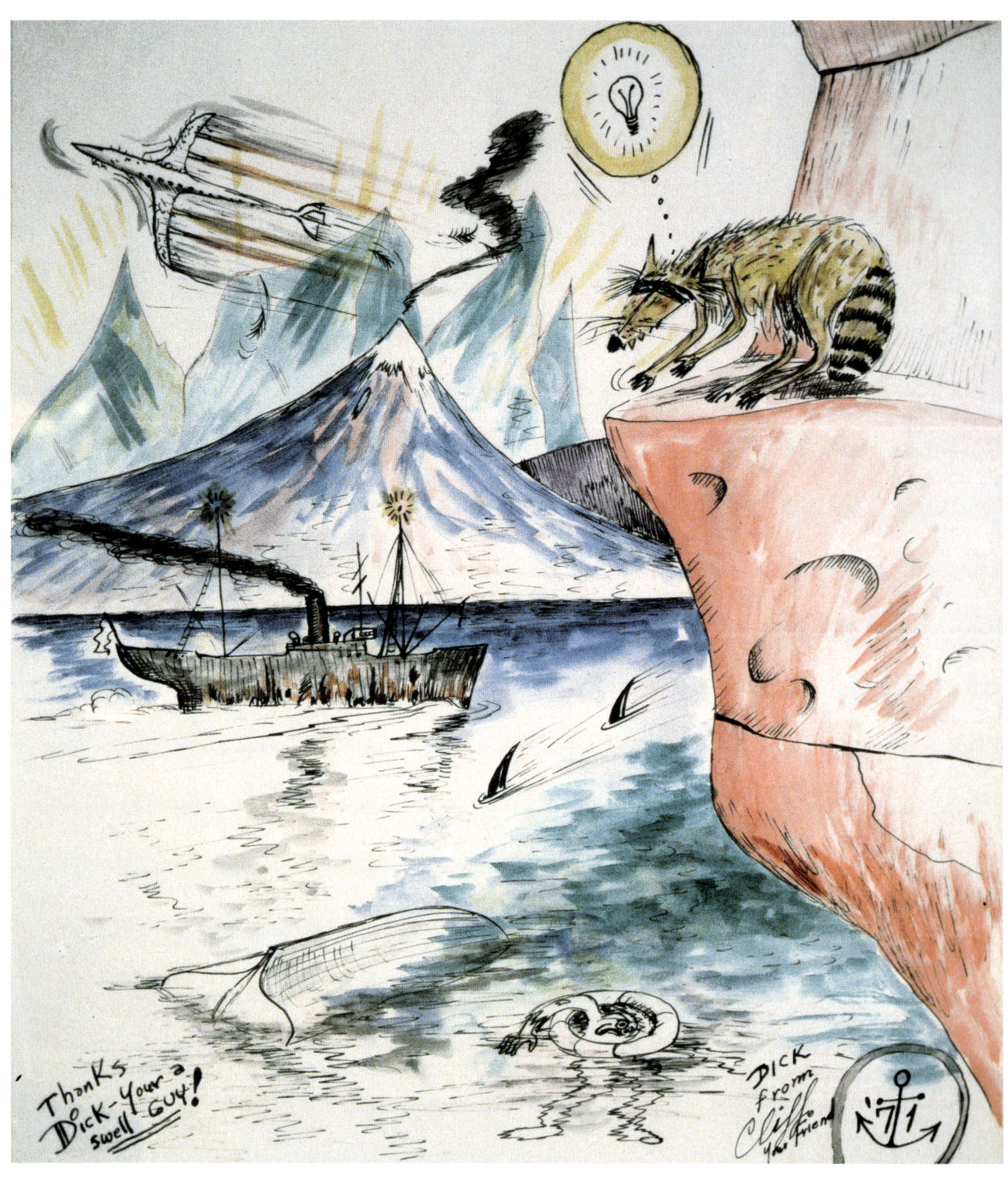
Thanks
Dick - Your a
swell GUY!
DICK
from
Cliff
Your Friend
'71

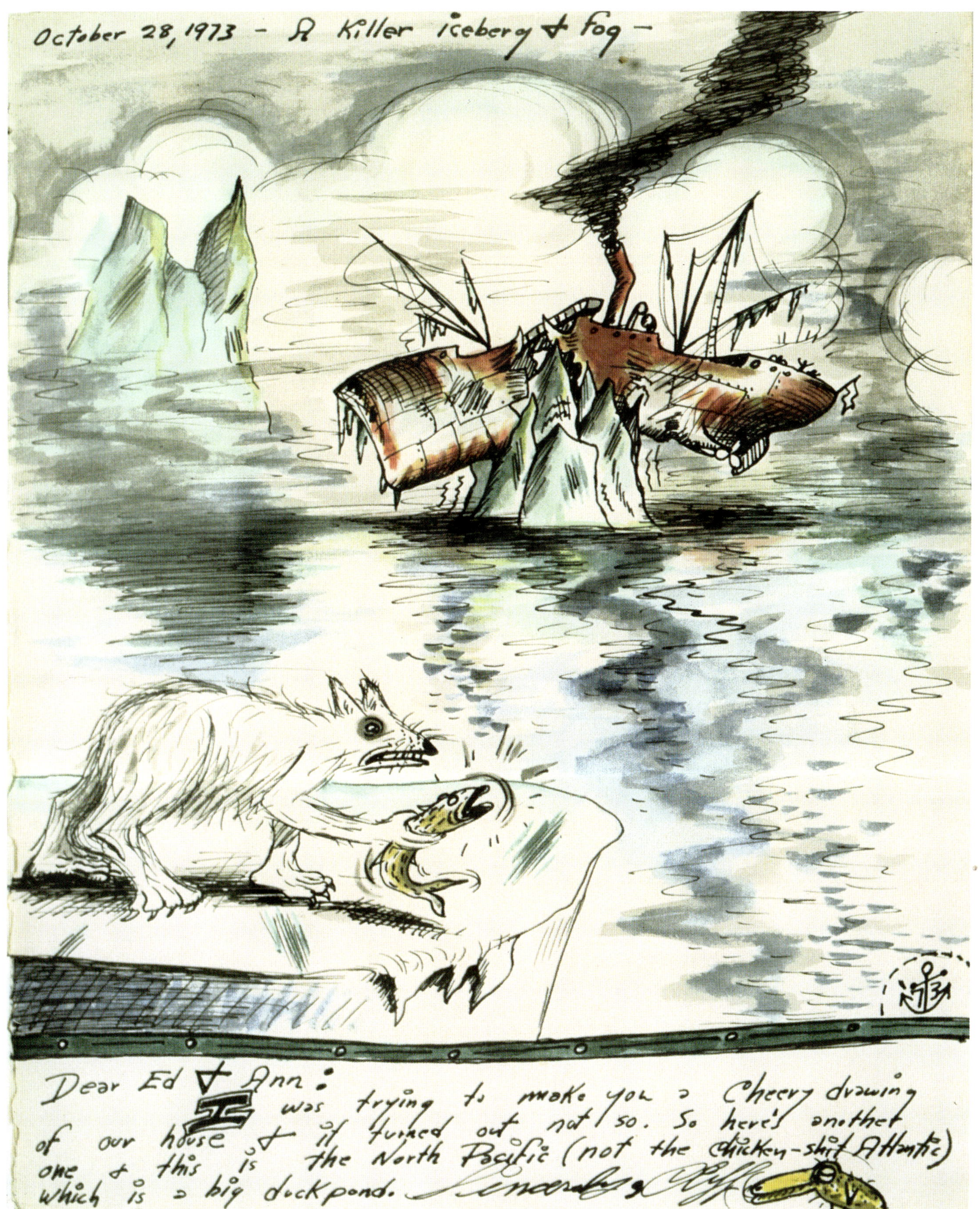
October 28, 1973 - A Killer iceberg & fog -
Dear Ed & Ann: I was trying to make you a cheery drawing
of our house & it turned out not so. So here's another
one & this is the North Pacific (not the chicken-shit Atlantic)
which is a big duckpond.

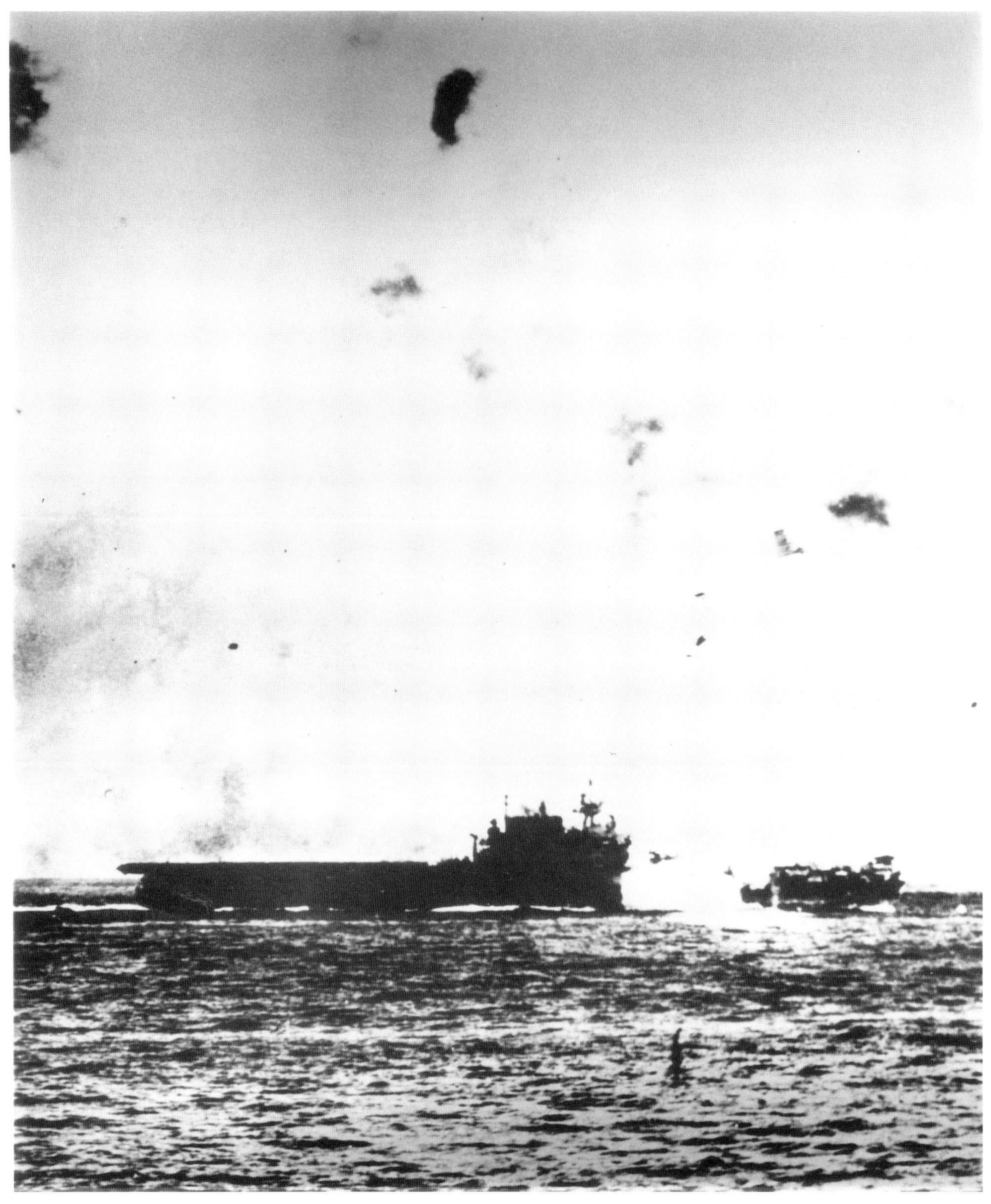

USS Enterprise during kamikaze attack, 1945

from a letter to Herk van Tongeren May 25, 1977

Right after WW II started I was stationed on the old "West Virginia" (a bird cage battlewagon) similar to the one in the postcard. The ship was hit badly at Pearl Harbor you know + I went on board just in time to help clean up all the shit + it was a mess allright. + one day working below decks they discovered in a watertight food locker some dead sailors that had plenty of food + they got air from a little vent that went up topside + had not been damaged. The West Virginia after it got hit just settled on the bottom of the harbor, right side up + was practically all underwater except for its superstructure. Well these sailors lived down there for 22 days, as they marked off the days on the bulkhead. What finally killed them was the fact that in raising it + cleaning debris they cut off their air supply, that vent. Unfortunately that was the end of those poor bastards. + in the clean up we used to find bones mixed in with the oil + parts of bodies etc. It was a shittin mess. Actually I was in the Marine detachment (80 of us) there + it was the most horse-shit rotten ship detachment in the whole fuckin Marine Corps + I finally got shit-canned thank God + went on the old Enterprise (a carrier) + it was great. I loved that ship + the detachment was OK too. Oh well Herk I shouldn't have gotten off on that crap. Anyway I sure appreciate your little gifts.

from a letter to Herk van Tongeren April 19, 1978

Once during the war (WW II that is) when I was stationed on the old Enterprise (carrier) we were out there in the Pacific so long that once I didn't step foot off it for a year + a half + then it was for a day on a working party on an ammunition ship. A few days later we left that atoll + we learned the ship had blown up. Naturally it completely disintegrated (the fate of an ammunition ship). I never quite forgot that + I don't know why I happened to mention that at this moment. Anyway the point of the story was that being on the Enterprise for that length of time didn't bother me at all. I loved that ship + the sea + about everything that went with it except for some of those Kamikaze attacks, etc. + just toward the end of the war we took a direct hit by one of those fuckers and had terrible casualties and damage. It was up forward just behind the #1 elevator + our engines + steering gear weren't fucked up so we were able to limp back to the States. I think we were one of the last ships hit by those frightening things. What they were was actually seeing death coming at you right down your fucking gun barrel + I was a gunner too all those years.

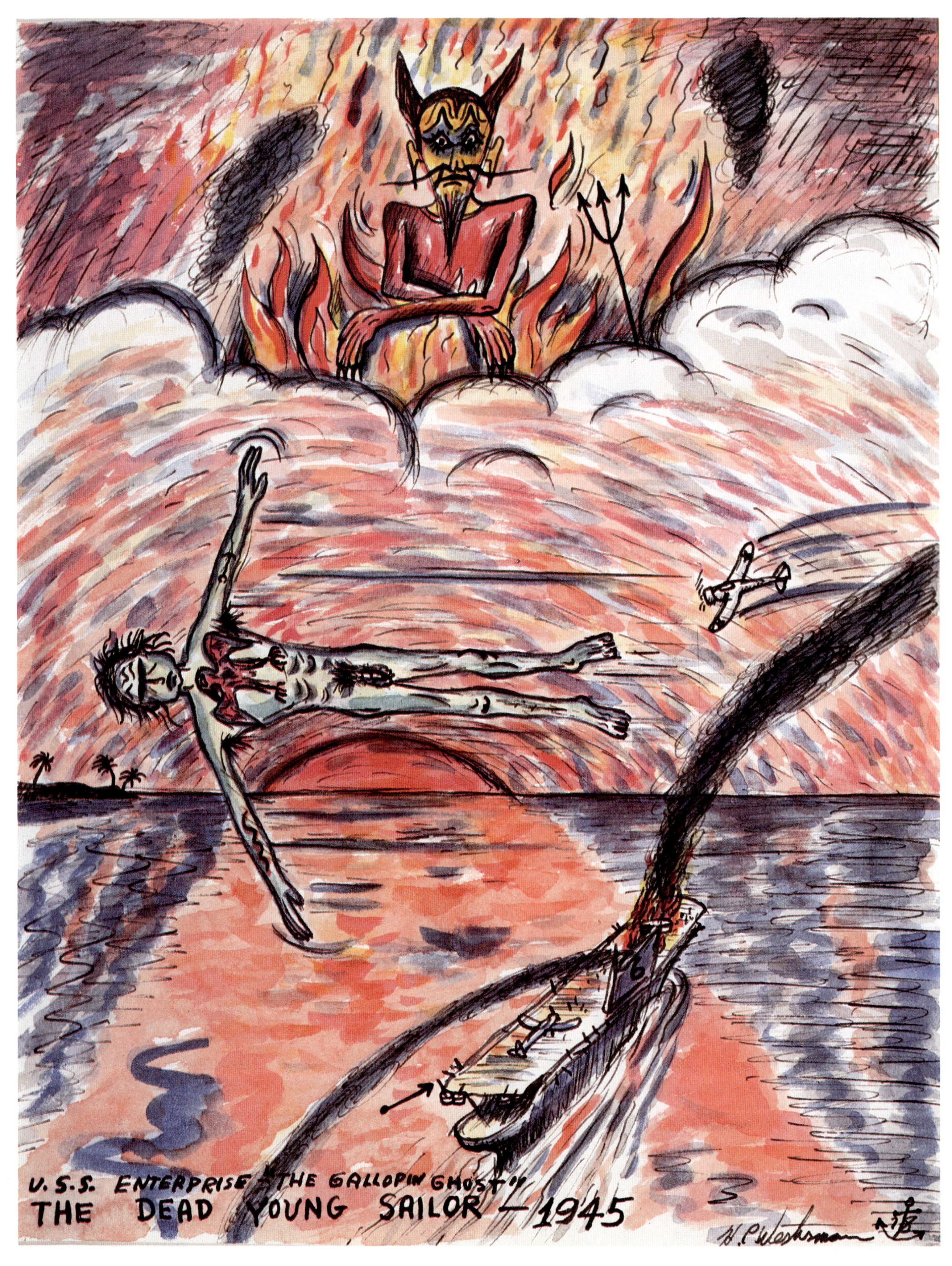
U.S.S. ENTERPRISE "THE GALLOPIN GHOST"
THE DEAD YOUNG SAILOR – 1945

May 3, 1978

Dear Tom:

It seems now to have evolved so quickly + now here it is practically time for the opening. Pretty exciting for me! Tom I'd like to say Barbara sent me a copy of her essay + I think it is excellent. She is 1st class — in fact I can't think of anyone I would rather have written the essay. As to the significance of the work — I think Barbara has an excellent grasp of it. The essay surprised me because of the seriousness, scholarly + perceptive quality of the composition. She really put a lot of thought into the work I have done + hence into her essay. There was nothing in it that I suggested she might delete or add or revise etc. She did a swell job! Tom, on behalf of the show I would like very much to personally thank you + whoever else was responsible for deciding on the show. I would like very much if some fine things would come of this show, for your museum — whatever that would be? Yours is a damn fine museum + I would like nothing better than to enhance it in some way!

About this drawing of the sailor — I'll try to explain it: This really happened — you see the little arrow in the drawing pointing to that after-gun. Well I was the gunner there of that time. One morning early a lone Japanese kamikaze attacked us from the rear at about a 45 degree angle. We knew it was a kamikaze immediately. All of us who could bear on the guy naturally fired at him when he came within range — I saw my tracers going into the god-damned thing but he kept coming down anyway (all this happened very fast). Well he hit up forward just aft of the # 1 elevator, which was up at the time + his plane exploded in the elevator pit. It blew our elevator 400 feet into the air (10 tons) + they don't know whether it was still going up or coming down when they snapped a photograph of it from another ship. Well it was a terrific explosion + many people up forward were killed + wounded + there was a terrific fire up there. They did get the fire put out finally + that night (+ it was a full moon). I was on watch back there on my gun position. I looked down on the fantail of the ship + they had all the dead people stacked there like cordwood. It was a pretty ungodly sight. Well the moon was bright + the dead sailor on top of the pile was a good pal of mine. That's him in the drawing. I recognized him immediately — he was naked + on his chest was a huge beautiful tattoo of an eagle that he was so proud of. In fact that tattoo hadn't quite been finished as we had to leave port suddenly a couple of years before. Well the next morning they placed each dead man in a mattress cover with a 5″ projectile tied between his legs + we buried them at sea. He was a very sweet guy. The best to you Tom + everybody involved with the show + my thanks.

Sincerely,
Cliff

Late Letters

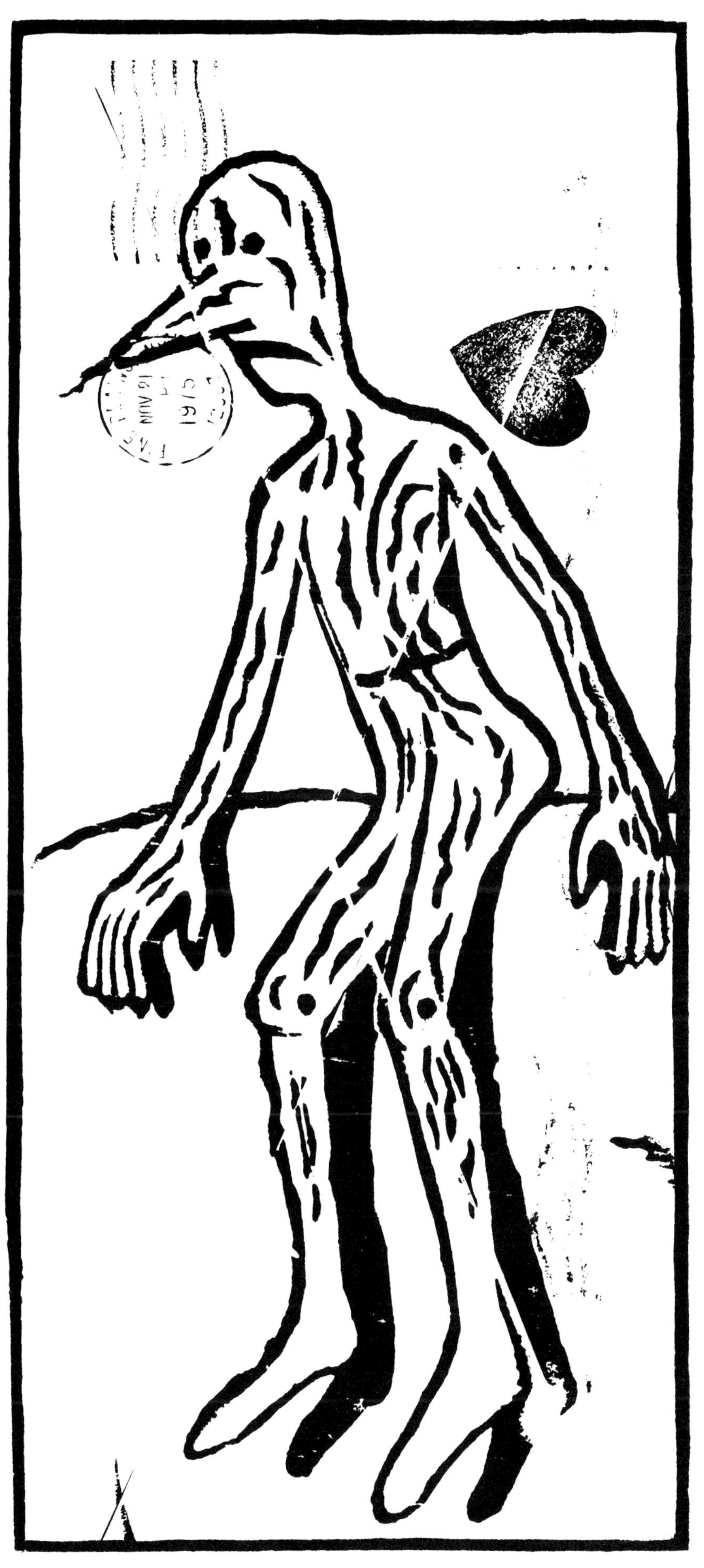

May 27, 1976

Dear Martha + Mike + Girls:

Do you realize, Martha, that you've been writing me consistently now for about 35 years. That is something! + that is a stack of letters that would stretch from here to the moon or fill up a gymnasium. Not only that but it sure has meant a lot to me over the years. Many times in the past a letter from you would arrive at a critical time + give me a shot in the arm just when it was needed. The power of a letter is incredible. Well I don't forget it Martha + I certainly have appreciated your taking the time to write. Dad was smart. Just before I went to Korea I visited them in Phoenix, you remember — + he sensed I was really low because Penny had taken off with the boy + that girl Mary. Well we went out for a walk + that's when he told me about being married once before + after only 2 weeks his new wife had taken off from him + he had searched frantically all over for her + nothing. I think that was in St. Louis? Well that must have been a shocker for him + I didn't feel so sorry for myself after that. I wonder who she was? Well anyway if she hadn't split you + La Nore + I wouldn't be here. So I'm all for it now + he is gone. So it doesn't make any difference. + Mother — she had that weird obsession about Annapolis, a really one track mind, but that's OK too. There's really nothing now for me to forgive — because it worked out OK + she is gone too, really long gone now! + Carl, it's like his father died yesterday — I don't think he ever got over that + you know he committed suicide in 1925 which was one hell of a long time ago. Families are weird + all life is so strange. The only thing that is real about the whole thing is that it is very short, right? Thank you for your last fine letter Martha + all my love.

Cliff

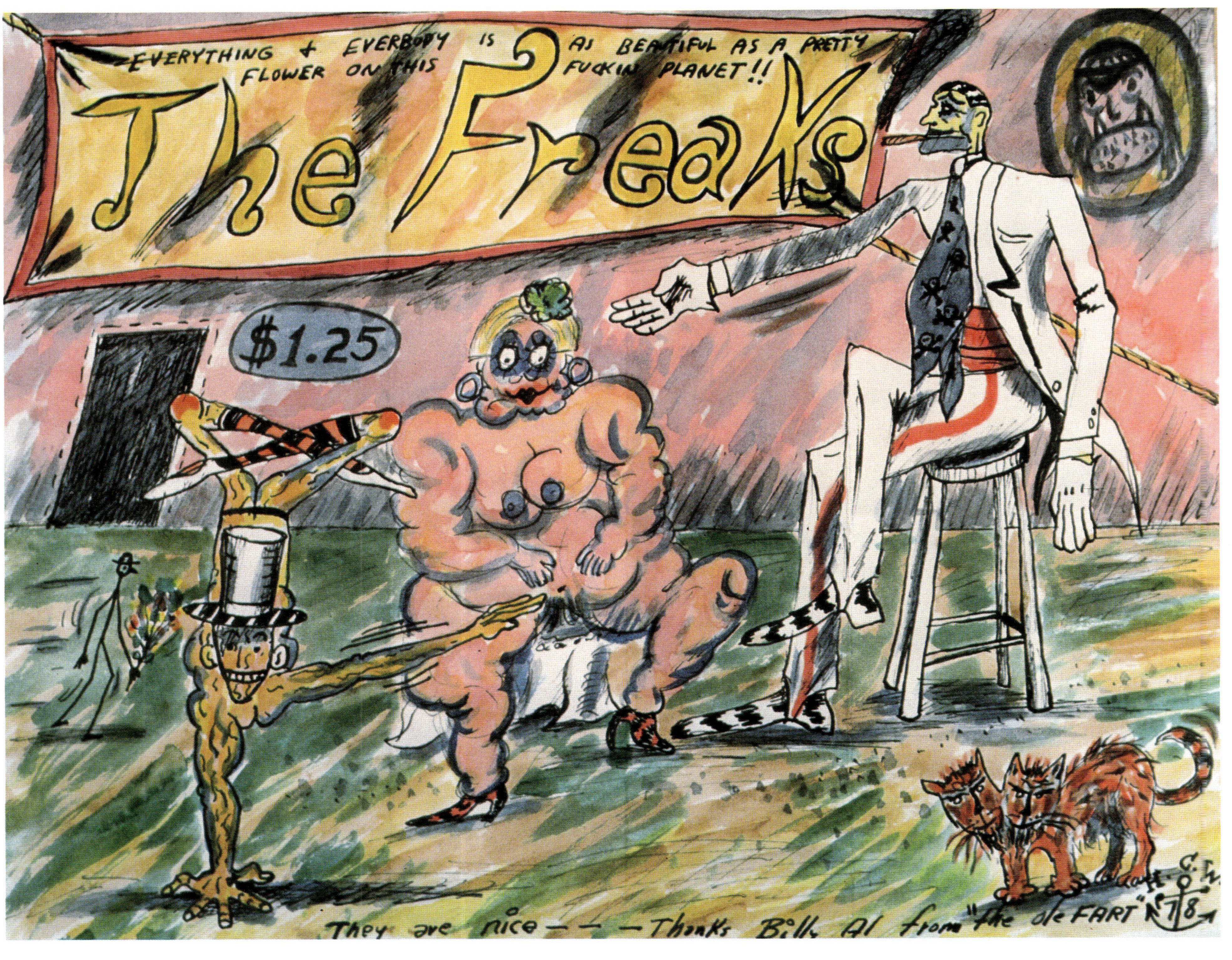
EVERYTHING + EVERBODY IS AS BEAUTIFUL AS A PRETTY FLOWER ON THIS FUCKIN PLANET!!
The Freaks
$1.25
They are nice - - - Thanks Billy Al from "the ole FART"
C.W.
78

March 22, 1978

Dear Bruce + Doris:

I been on ice here in the shit house for one month today (+ I'm going home Fri. + I'm walking out). I'll explain this in a minute. Since I was able I've been thinking a lot about both of you — + in particular how knowing you, all these years has meant so much to me + when I think about you — it always makes me feel real good + cheers me up. There have never been very God damned many people I have met in my life that have really impressed me so. Joanny, of course, has always really turned me on. But other than Joanny + you two + a couple of others + that's about it. Well back to why I'm here ------- I helped all winter getting us through the fuckin blizzards + I never saw so much snow + ice in my life. Well towards the end of it all (a month ago) I had to turn into the hospital here because I have this fucking physical problem. Once I got in I guess I lost my grip + had a mother-fucking heart attack + my luck ran out. If I had had the thing at home I probably would have been a dead fucker. Anyway I'm convalescing real well + as I said they're letting me go Fri. (by the time you receive this letter). Joanny, luckily, has been staying with friends in N.Y. here + comes every day (she's a honey + gets finer all the time). Oddly enough, in spite of all these lousy problems, the Doc says I've got one damned good heart + I'm a good healer. I feel swell now but sure am looking forward to Friday! + of course I got to be damned careful now for a long time. Oh sure I can attend the opening + it's on May 17th — but I sure gotta take it easy. In the fall, perhaps, if I'm strong enough I've got to then have a big kidney operation, which will be a big deal I guess? One of the fuckers is dead + they're going to remove it — the other one is good but is only getting 20% of the blood it needs. It's a strange thing but I was born like this (inherited) + finally now they're going to fix it + the Doc says I'll be like a new man. The way I see it I'm God damned lucky to be able to walk out of here Fri. + go home. This letter's a lousy drag isn't it — I mean all this shit about my problems + hell everybody's got, usually, terrible problems, in one form or another. Somehow I feel like one of the lucky ones though. Well I'd like to apologize + perhaps I shouldn't even have written this God-damned thing? I'll never know. But, as I said I've been thinking a lot about you + your remarkable kids. I'd like to meet them some day. This letter is not meant to be complaining — I've had my share of luck + much more in this fucking life + I know it. I want you to know I always hope for the best for all of you + thanks very much for the past incredible memories.

Love,
Cliff

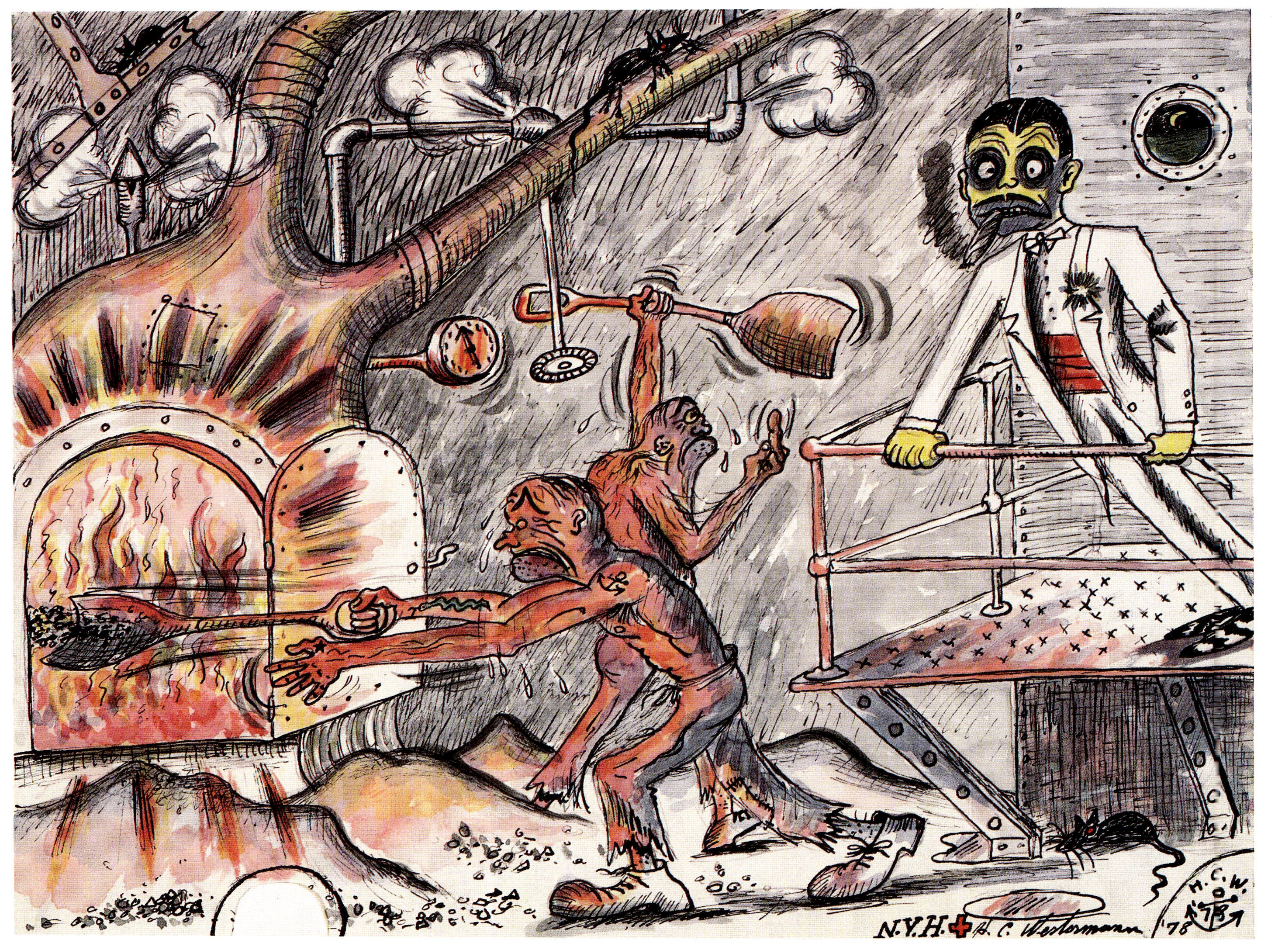
N.Y.H.
H.C. Westermann '78
H.C.W.

March 28, 1978

Dear Tom:

I'd like to try + explain all this bullshit — I mean these peculiar little drawings. Well I love to draw, you know, but I never keep them for myself. Oh sure I have given a lot of them to "the little flower" (my true love) otherwise I send them on — to interesting people (+ they are a substitute for a letter, which comes more difficult for me) + to people I like. I like your style Tom + you run a swell store. I mean the Whitney is First Class + on a high level + it is interesting! My favorite place + I'm sure a lot of artists share that sentiment. Somehow I feel as though I know you, to a certain degree (perhaps because of your museum?) On the other hand the M.O.M.A. is a disappointment. They ruined a beautiful building first + their concept is peculiar. For instance I saw the Cezanne show there + they did that fine, fine artist a disservice. For one thing it reminded me of a kindergarten class for children on art ("Now children do this + do that + look at this + one + one is two, etc"). Poor ole Cezanne would have turned over in his fuckin grave! Perhaps you've heard I was on ice for a month + it was serious Tom — I never thought I'd make it this time — but I'm home now + I feel great, am convalescing + getting stronger everyday + the Doc says I certainly may attend the opening on May 17th. Thanks again Tom + keep up the fine work.

Respectfully,
Cliff

We'll have a party when
I get home - A great party - OH - BOY!

Sure do
miss you!

Love

Cliff

NYH

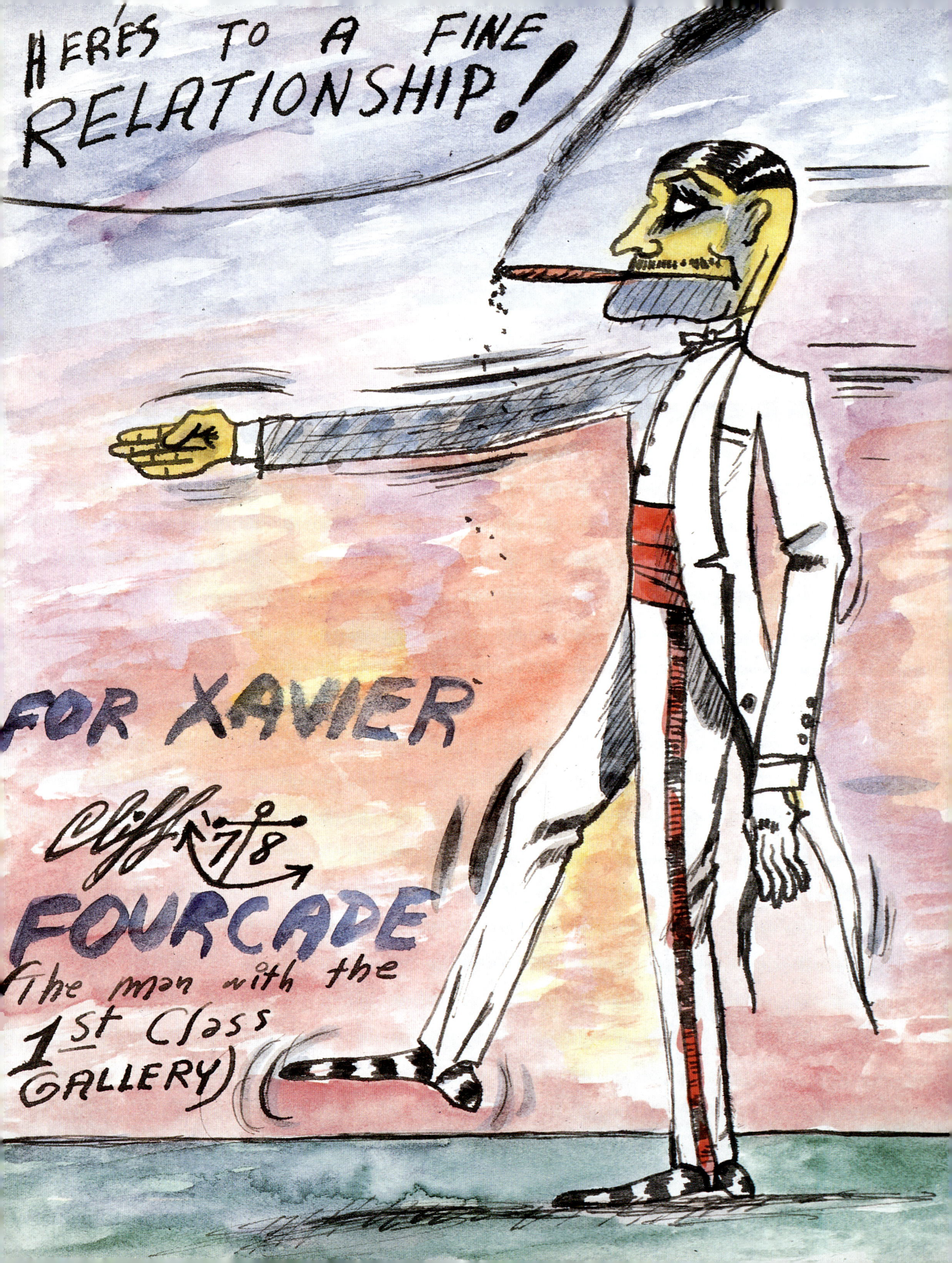
HERE'S TO A FINE RELATIONSHIP!
FOR XAVIER
Cliff 7/8
FOURCADE
(The man with the 1st Class GALLERY)

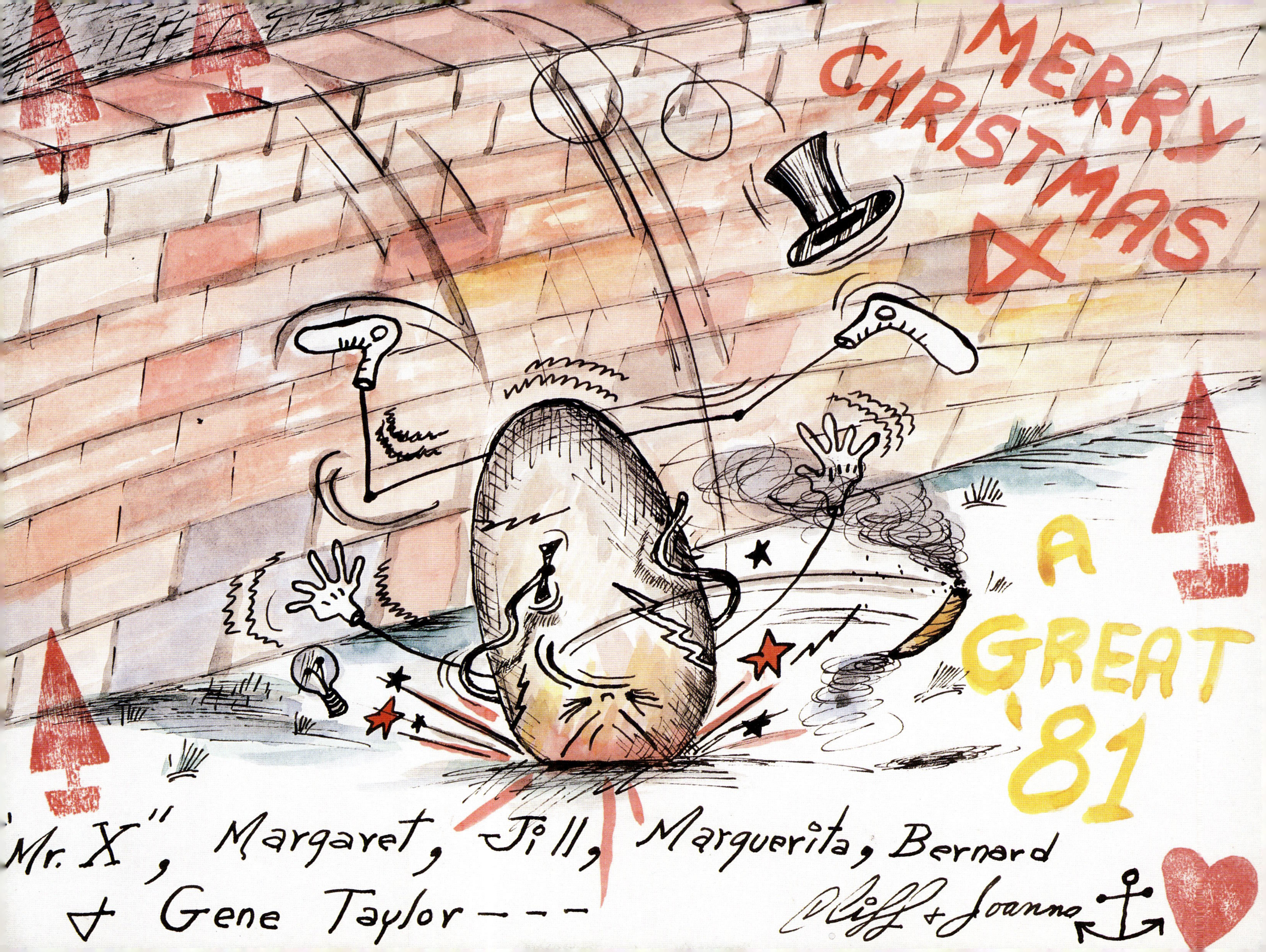
MERRY CHRISTMAS
A GREAT '81
"Mr. X", Margaret, Jill, Marguerita, Bernard
+ Gene Taylor---
Cliff + Joanna

September 17, 1981

Dear Terry + Jo Harvey:

The only good thing I've heard on the radio in the last 25 years is that now the bright boys have concluded that a little alcohol is very good for you. It stimulates + enhances the action of the heart. All the rest of the bull-shit, over the air, forget it. + oh yeh the only good thing the Gov't has done since Thomas Jefferson was to make this rose stamp on this envelope + I chalk that one up to some kind of a mistake. Anyway it's not a bad rose. Gee I want to thank you for your last snappy letter + postcard. I assume with all of your traveling Terry you mean you have been doing club dates with your band? Jo Harvey, we have yet to have had the pleasure of seeing and hearing one of your performances + we are still looking forward to that. So many people who saw your one in N.Y. have told us how terrific it was. I wish we had seen it. You know after getting a lot of catalogs of shows, from all over the country, I am convinced there is a lot of real terrific ART being done nowadays — + all over the country. I am truly amazed, so many people sincerely trying desperately to do genuine expressions. That makes me feel real good. In fact there's a lot of marvelous people running around out there. Unfortunately none of them are in Gov't, etc. + the museums + the institutions are kind of fucked up. But people — WOW — they are something else, particularly Artists. You know, Terry, when we hear Juarez (+ we appreciate it + love it more all the time) I still cry, usually — it sure gets to us. + boy oh boy how I love the raunchy Lubbock woman + Joe Bob, + the other ones. I often wonder where the New Delhi express ended up. I used to ride the freights, on the West coast, when I was a kid + got fucked up in a few of those hobo jungles + finally learned to stay clear of them + their 25 cent a gallon rot gut. My gouty son, you know the guy in the Air Force, on Okinawa, well he's still a mess + is trying to drink all the coffee (35 cups a day) from one end of the Island to the other, + smoke up all their cigarettes. He's still got 2 1/2 years to do on that lousy rock. The thing is I love the lousy mother-fucker, + he's the only son I got + underneath he's got good things going for him. It's just that lousy war that turned him inside out + scrambled his brains. I'm amazed the Air Force has let him stay in + hasn't given him a goofy discharge. He can't do a fucking thing, which is OK by me + he's got a funny wife — I mean she's a fireball + the best thing going for her is that she's a Texas girl + anyone from Texas just can't be too wrong. That's still our favorite place. Unfortunately we haven't been able to get back there since that last time + my doctor has got me back in the sack again for I don't know how long. Overwork or something this time. I can get out of the sack + go piss or sit down once in a while to write a letter. Nothing serious, but fuck it + I gotta eat that shit-eating baby food etc. When Joanny goes out someplace in the truck though I dive out of the sack + head for the refrigerator + grab a beer + down the fucker bottle + all in about 3 seconds + smoke a half dozen cigars. Oh well bull shit you can't hang in there forever + that's OK with me. "Let the chips fall where they want to".

Cliff

EARLY LETTERS

Tattooed Chest *(page 15)*, undated, ink on paper, 6 1/4 x 9 1/2, collection Martha Renner

When Horace comes marching home *(page 16)*, circa 1943, ink on onion skin, 11 7/8 x 9 1/8, collection Martha Renner

Post War Plans *(page 17)*, 1945, ink on paper, 9 1/2 x 6 1/4, collection Martha Renner

Wayne and Westermann — Handbalancers *(page 18)*, 1946, ink on paper, 13 13/16 x 11 9/16, collection Martha Renner

(page 19) photograph of Westermann handbalancing with Bill Lichtenwalter on the USS Enterprise in 1944 with an excerpt from a letter to Barbara Haskell, written January 11, 1978, to clarify some points regarding Cliff's biography

Happy Fathers Day *(page 20)*, 1949, ink and watercolor on paper, 12 1/2 x 18 1/4, collection Martha Renner

(page 21) unillustrated letter to Martha and Mike Renner, October 14, 1976

Champion of Justice *(page 22)*, circa 1959, ink and watercolor on paper, 13 1/2 x 10 5/8, sent to Allan Frumkin, private collection, New York

(page 23) unillustrated letter to Martha and Mike Renner, September 20, 1958

The Smoker *(page 24)*, circa 1959, ink and watercolor on paper, 13 1/2 x 10 5/8, sent to Allan Frumkin, private collection, New York

Cliff carving a portrait of Allan Frumkin *(page 25)*, 1961, pen and ink on paper, 13 3/8 x 10 1/2, sent to Allan Frumkin, private collection, New York

(page 26) photograph of Westermann in his studio at 222 North Avenue, Chicago, 1960, photograph by Philip Fantl

(page 27) unillustrated letter to Martha and Mike Renner, February 24, 1959

Astronaut *(page 28)*, 1962, ink on paper, 12 1/16 x 9, sent to Allan Frumkin private collection, New York

Help $ *(page 29)*, 7/29/63, ink and watercolor on paper, 11 1/4 x 10 5/8, sent to Allan Frumkin, private collection, New York

Fall in Connecticut *(page 30)*, 1963, ink on paper, 11 15/16 x 8 15/16 sent to Richard Hollander, collection the Spencer Museum of Art, University of Kansas, Lawrence, Kansas, anonymous gift

(page 31) unillustrated letter to Martha and Mike Renner, April 27, 1964

TRIBUTE TO AMERICA

The Great Mojave *(page 33)*, 1964, ink on paper, 12 x 17 5/8, sent to Allan Frumkin, private collection, New York

The Batmobile *(page 34)*, 7/25/64, ink and watercolor on paper, 10 3/4 x 14, collection Noma Copley

(page 35) photograph of Westermann in front of the batmobile in Los Angeles, 1964, with an excerpt from a letter to Allan Frumkin, June 29, 1964

Seneca State Park, W. Va. *(page 36)*, 8/26/64, ink on paper, 13 1/2 x 10 1/2, sent to Allan Frumkin, private collection, New York

Pinesville, KY *(page 37)*, 8/29/64, ink on paper, 13 1/2 x 10 1/2, sent to Allan Frumkin, private collection, New York

Murfreesboro, Tenn. *(page 38)*, 9/1/64, ink on paper, 13 1/2 x 10 1/2, sent to Allan Frumkin, private collection, New York

Jackson, Tenn. *(page 39)*, 9/1/64, ink on paper, 10 1/2 x 13 1/2, sent to Allan Frumkin, private collection, New York

Muskogee, Okla. *(page 40)*, 9/4/64, ink on paper, 13 1/2 x 10 1/2, sent to Allan Frumkin, private collection, New York

N. Tex. *(page 41)*, 9/6/64, ink on paper, 10 1/2 x 13 1/2, sent to Allan Frumkin, private collection, New York

N.M. *(page 42)*, 9/8/64, ink on paper, 10 1/2 x 13 1/2, sent to Allan Frumkin, private collection, New York

Near Cuba, N.M. *(page 43)*, 9/9/64, watercolor and ink on paper, 11 5/8 x 16, sent to Allan Frumkin, private collection, New York

Tuba City, Arizona *(page 44)*, 9/10/64, ink on paper, 11 1/2 x 16 1/8, sent to Allan Frumkin, private collection, New York

L.A. *(page 45)*, 9/15/64, ink on paper, 13 1/2 x 10 1/2, sent to Dot and Lester Beall, collection Joanna Beall Westermann

U.S.A. *(page 46)*, 1964, ink and watercolor on paper, 13 7/8 x 16 3/4, sent to Allan Frumkin, private collection, New York

Madame Butterfly *(page 47)*, 1965, ink and watercolor on paper, 13 7/8 x 16 3/4, collection Joanna Beall Westermann

SCULPTURE

Cliff made out of tools *(page 49)*, 1959, ink on paper, 9 3/8 x 6 3/8, collection Joanna Beall Westermann

Mysteriously Abandoned New Home *(page 50)*, 1958, ink and watercolor on paper, 13 1/2 x 10 1/2, collection Joanna Beall Westermann

(page 51) excerpts from two unillustrated letters to Martha and Mike Renner: 1959 and 2/27/64

Plush *(page 52)*, 1963, ink and watercolor on paper, 11 7/8 x 8 3/4, sent to Allan Frumkin, private collection, New York

Family Tree *(page 53)*, 2/14/64, ink and watercolor on paper, 8 7/8 x 11 7/8, sent to Allan Frumkin, private collection, New York

Suicide *(page 54)*, 2/26/64, ink and watercolor on paper, 11 3/4 x 8 7/8, sent to Allan Frumkin, private collection, New York

Social Problems *(page 55)*, second page of the above letter

Idea of a Brand New City *(pages 56 and 57)*, 3/16/64, ink and watercolor on paper, 13 3/4 x 10 3/4, sent to Allan Frumkin, private collection, New York

Aluminated *(pages 58 and 59)*, 1964, ink and watercolor on paper, 11 7/8 x 8 7/8, sent to Allan Frumkin, private collection, New York

Four Wood Reliefs *(page 61)*, 2/17/65, ink on paper, 13 1/2 x 10 1/2, *(page 60)* excerpt from the above letter, sent to Allan Frumkin, private collection, New York

The Fourteenth Wood Relief *(page 62)* and ***The Slob*** *(page 63)*, 3/5/65, ink on paper, 13 5/8 x 10 3/8, sent to Allan Frumkin, private collection, New York

A Piece from the Museum of Shattered Dreams *(page 64)*, 4/5/65, pen and ink on paper, 14 1/8 x 16 3/4, sent to Allan Frumkin, private collection, New York

The Museum Piece, Pacific Miss and another Plaque *(page 65)*, 4/17/65, ink and watercolor on paper, second page of a letter to Allan Frumkin, 16 5/8 x 13 7/8, private collection, New York

Nowhere *(pages 66 and 67)*, 6/1/65, ink on paper, a three page letter to Allan Frumkin, 10 5/8 x 13 1/2, private collection, New York, with excerpt from a letter to Barbara Haskell 10/30/77 referring to the drawing of *The Little Black Cage*

Homage to American Art *(page 68)*, 3/28/66, ink and watercolor on paper, 13 1/2 x 10, sent to Allan Frumkin, private collection, New York

Death Ship run over by a Lincoln Continental *(page 69)*, 9/27/66, ink and watercolor on paper, 9 3/4 x 13 1/2, sent to Allan Frumkin, private collection, New York

Death Ship of No Port *(page 70)*, 1/6/67, ink on paper, 13 1/2 x 10 5/8, sent to Allan Frumkin, private collection, New York

I Made a Deal with God *(page 71)*, 3/16/68, ink and watercolor on paper, 13 1/2 x 10 1/2, sent to Allan Frumkin, private collection, New York

(page 72) unillustrated letter to Allan Frumkin, 10/20/69

(page 73) unillustrated letter to Allan Frumkin, 11/4/76

Aluminum Hands *(pages 74 and 75)*, 12/28/78, sent to Richard Hollander, ink and watercolor on paper, 13 3/16 x 9 5/16, collection the Spencer Art Museum, University of Kansas, Lawrence, Kansas, anonymous gift

The Man from the Torrid Zone *(pages 76 and 77)*, 1980-81, pen and ink on paper, 12 x 9, letter addressed to Xavier Fourcade, collection Gilbert Kinney

JOANNA

Note: all the letters in this section are in the collection of Joanna Beall Westermann

Beautiful Joanna *(page 79)*, 10/17/68, ink on paper, detail from a letter, 11 x 8 1/2

Valentine *(page 80)*, 1960, ink and watercolor on paper, 13 1/2 x 10 3/4

Dear Lop Lop *(page 81)*, 5/16/61, ink, watercolor and newspaper on paper, 13 1/2 x 10 3/4

Dear Mrs. Sweeda beed A *(pages 82 and 83)*, 1961, ink on paper, 13 1/2 x 10

(page 84) photograph of Joanna Beall Westermann, 1962, photograph taken by H.C. Westermann, with excerpt from a letter to Dorothy and Lester Beall, Joanna's parents

Happy Birthday *(page 85)*, 1966, ink and watercolor on paper, 13 1/2 x 9 7/8

(page 86) photograph of Cliff, 1962, taken by Joanna Beall Westermann

Hi Ya Sweetheart *(page 87)*, 1968, ink on paper, 10 3/4 x 8 1/4

Honey *(page 88)*, 1967, ink and watercolor on paper, 13 3/4 x 10 1/2

(pages 89 and 90) four unillustrated letters, all written in 1968 while Westermann was at Tamarind in Los Angeles

Dearest Sweety *(page 91)*, April 1971, ink on paper, 10 x 8

Happy Valentines Joanny Dear *(page 92)*, 1977, ink and watercolor on paper, 9 3/8 x 13 3/4

Lilinonah *(page 93)*, 1978, ink and watercolor on paper, 9 x 12

A COUNTRY GONE NUTS

Airplane and Building *(page 95)*, 1962, woodcut print, 12 x 8 15/16, sent to Richard Hollander, collection Spencer Museum of Art, University of Kansas, Lawrence, Kansas, anonymous donation

Crimson Rose Building *(page 96)*, 1963, ink and watercolor on paper, 11 3/4 x 8 7/8, sent to Jean Frumkin, private collection, New York

Apathy *(page 97)*, 1963, pen and ink on paper, 12 x 9, sent to Allan Frumkin, private collection, New York

Goldwater–San Francisco *(page 98)*, 1964, pen and ink on paper, 11 3/4 x 17 3/4, sent to Allan Frumkin, private collection, New York

GOP Convention *(page 99)*, 1964, pen and ink on paper, 15 x 16 7/8, sent to Allan Frumkin with excerpt from an unillustrated letter to Allan Frumkin, 6/29/64, private collection, New York

Wm. Bonney *(page 100)*, 1964, pen and ink on paper, 12 x 17 5/8, sent to Allan Frumkin, private collection, New York

Poison Prunes *(page 101)*, 1965, pen and ink on paper, 14 x 16 3/4, collection Joanna Beall Westermann

Suicide Rehearsal *(pages 102 and 103)*, newspaper clipping, with Westermann's illustration of the event on the facing page, 1965, ink and watercolor on paper, 16 1/2 x 13 3/4, sent to Allan Frumkin, private collection, New York

Great Cultural Explosion *(page 104)*, 1966, ink on paper, 13 1/2 x 9 7/8, collection Dennis Adrian

He's Lost Interest in Us *(page 105)*, 1966, ink on paper, 13 3/8 x 10 1/4, collection Dennis Adrian

A Country Gone Nuts *(page 106)*, 10/4/66, ink and watercolor on paper, 13 1/2 x 9 7/8, sent to Allan Frumkin, private collection, New York

Poor Spec *(page 107)*, 1966, ink and watercolor on paper, 8 x 10, collection William Wiley

There are some men in this country *(page 108)*, 6/17/68, ink on paper, 13 1/2 x 10 1/2, sent to William Copley, collection Billy Copley

Stop the War *(page 109)*, 1973, ink on paper, 5 3/4 x 10, collection Joanna Beall Westermann with an excerpt of a letter to Bruce and Doris Oxford, 3/29/78

Muhammed Ali Fight *(page 110)*, 1976, newspaper, ink and watercolor on paper, 10 x 8, collection Al Shean

Who Flung Dung *(page 111)*, 1977, newspaper, pen and ink on paper, 10 x 8, collection Robert and Mavis Hudson

FRIENDS

The Handshake *(page 113)*, mid-1970s, ink on paper, 8 x 10, from a letter to Joanna Beall Westermann

Hearts of Gold *(page 114)*, 1965/6, ink and watercolor on paper, 13 1/2 x 10 1/8, collection Dennis Adrian

Elasticity of Old Age *(page 115)*, 1965/6, ink and watercolor on paper, 9 x 6 1/4, collection Dennis Adrian

Sharks Eating Artists and a Tribute to Dennis *(page 116)*, 8/5/65, ink and watercolor on paper, 10 1/2 x 13 1/2, collection Robert and Rhett Delford Brown

Dear Richard Thank You *(page 117)*, 9/27/66, ink, watercolor and a dollar bill on paper, 13 1/2 x 9 7/16, letter sent to Richard Hollander, collection Spencer Museum of Art, University of Kansas, Lawrence, Kansas, anonymous gift

From the Road Apple *(page 118)*, 1967, ink and cigar label on paper, 10 1/2 x 7 1/4, collection Ken Price

Te Amo is my favorite cigar *(page 119)*, 12/6/68, ink on paper, 11 x 8 1/2, letter to Allan Frumkin, private collection, New York

The Human Fly *(page 120)*, 1971, ink and watercolor on paper 10 5/8 x 8, collection Noma Copley

The Witch *(page 121)*, 10/31/72, ink on paper, 10 1/2 x 7 1/4, sent to Ed and Sarah Flood, collection Cheryl Flood

Cliff in Tails *(page 122)*, 3/18/72, ink and watercolor on paper, 16 1/2 x 13 1/4, collection Ed Ruscha

Cliff losing his teeth *(page 123)*, 11/2/72, ink on paper, 16 5/8 x 13 3/4, collection Al Shean

Sailboat *(page 124)*, 3/15/72, ink and watercolor on paper, 9 3/4 x 7 3/4, collection Robert and Rhett Delford Brown, with an excerpt from a letter to Roger Brouard, 1981

Welcome Home *(page 125)*, 1974 or 1975, ink and watercolor on paper, 10 1/4 x 8, addressed to Ed and Sarah Flood, collection Cheryl Flood

(page 126) letter sent to Dr. Laragh, Columbia Presbyterian Hospital, 1974

Dog and Santa *(page 127)*, 1975, ink and watercolor on paper, 13 7/8 x 11, collection Mike Nevelson

Cliff as Bartender *(page 128)*, 1976, ink on paper, 11 x 14, collection James Corcoran

An Old Sea Hag *(page 129)*, 2/9/77, ink and watercolor on paper, 8 3/4 x 12, collection Ed Janss

The Great Escape from Block Island *(page 130)*, 1/4/78, ink and watercolor on paper, 8 5/8 x 11 with excerpt from the rest of the letter, collection Mavis and Robert Hudson

Terry Allen Composer *(page 131)*, 1980, 8 1/2 x 11, with an excerpt from a letter to Terry and Jo Harvey Allen 6/5/79, collection Terry and Jo Harvey Allen

BROOKFIELD CENTER

(page 133) photograph of the rafters of the house in Brookfield Center taken by H.C. Westermann

Brookfield Center *(page 134)*, 10/12/65, ink and watercolor on decorated card, 11 x 8 1/2, collection Martha Renner

(page 135) excerpts from letters to: Bruce and Doris Oxford, 12/27/67; Herk and Diane van Tongeren, 11/4/71; Martha and Mike Renner, 9/3/81

(page 136) photograph of H.C. Westermann taken by Joanna Beall Westermann, 1971

(page 137) photograph of the entrance to the house taken by Bill Barrette, 1987

Yeah *(page 138)*, 1972, ink and watercolor on paper, 11 x 8 1/2, collection Joanna Beall Westermann

Pale Horse and Rider *(page 139)*, 10/13/73, ink and watercolor on paper, 13 3/4 x 11, collection Ed Janss

Cliff and Joanna working on their house *(page 140)*, 7/9/69, ink on paper, 8 1/2 x 11, collection Billy Al Bengston and photograph of Joanna's studio below, taken by Bill Barrette, 1987

Cliff the Ranger *(page 141)*, 1977, ink on paper, 9 1/4 x 12 1/4, collection Jerry Ordover and photograph of Westermann's studio and house taken by Bill Barrette, 1987

Cliff killing gypsy moths *(page 142)*, 6/21/81, last page of a letter to Gene Bowen, ink on paper, 8 1/2 x 11, letter printed in full above drawing

(page 143) photograph of Westermann on his front porch, summer of 1981, photograph taken by Bobbe Wolfe

(page 144) photograph of Westermann's studio taken by Bill Barrette, 1987

(page 145) unillustrated letter to Ruth Marchant, Westermann's aunt, 10/30/81

DEATH SHIPS

USS Enterprise *(page 147)*, 1959?, ink on paper, 8 1/2 x 11, letter to Allan Frumkin, private collection, New York

Early Death Ship *(page 148)*, 1959, ink on paper, 11 x 8 1/2, letter to Allan Frumkin, private collection, New York

(page 149) unillustrated letter to Herk van Tongeren, 4/14/71

Ship as Skyscraper *(page 150)*, 1965, pen and ink on paper, 16 5/8 x 14, letter to Allan Frumkin, private collection, New York

Terrifying Sea Picture *(page 151)*, 1966, pen and ink on paper, 13 1/2 x 9 7/8, letter to Allan Frumkin, private collection, New York

Death Ship USS Franklin *(page 152)*, 1966, ink and watercolor on paper, 13 1/2 x 9 7/8, collection Dennis Adrian

Odyssey *(page 153)*, 11/8/66, ink on paper, 13 1/2 x 10, collection Noma Copley

Same drawing I love to do *(page 154)*, 1966, ink and watercolor on paper, 13 1/2 x 9 7/8, letter to Jean Frumkin, private collection, New York

Port of Shadows *(page 155)*, 1966, ink on paper, 13 1/2 x 9 7/8, letter to Allan Frumkin, private collection, New York

Ship in the Woods with Sharks *(page 156)*, 10/31/69, ink on paper, 7 1/4 x 10 3/4, letter to Allan Frumkin, private collection, New York

Obituary for Frank *(page 157)*, 12/10/71, ink and newspaper on paper, 7 7/8 x 10 3/4, letter to Allan Frumkin, private collection, New York

Raccoon with Death Ship *(page 158)*, 1971, ink and watercolor on paper, 16 5/8 x 13 15/16, collection Richard Riesman

A Killer Iceberg *(page 159)*, 10/28/73, ink and watercolor on paper, 11 x 14, collection Ed Janss

(page 160) photograph of USS Enterprise and kamikaze attack, 1945

(page 161) excerpts from letters to Herk van Tongeren, 5/25/77 and 4/19/78

The Dead Young Sailor — 1945 *(page 162 and 163)*, 5/3/78, ink and watercolor on paper, 11 7/8 x 8 7/8, with letter to Thomas N. Armstrong, III, collection Whitney Museum of American Art, New York

LATE LETTERS

Pinocchio *(page 165)*, 1976, woodcut on paper, 9 3/8 x 4 11/16, sent to Richard Hollander, collection Spencer Museum of Art, University of Kansas, Lawrence, Kansas

(page 166) unillustrated letter to Martha and Mike Renner, 5/27/76

The Freaks *(page 167)*, 1978, ink and watercolor on paper, 8 7/8 x 11 7/8, collection Billy Al Bengston

The Furnace *(page 168)*, 1978, ink and watercolor on paper, 9 x 12, collection Joanna Beall Westermann

(page 169) unillustrated letter to Bruce and Doris Oxford, 3/22/78

(page 170) unillustrated letter to Thomas N. Armstrong, III, 3/28/78, Whitney Museum of American Art

Sure Do Miss You *(page 171)*, 1978, ink on paper, 10 x 8, collection Joanna Beall Westermann

Here's to a Fine Relationship *(page 172)*, 1978, ink and watercolor on paper, 9 3/4 x 8 1/2, collection Xavier Fourcade

Humpty Dumpty *(page 173)*, 1980, ink and watercolor on paper, 9 x 12, collection Xavier Fourcade

(page 174) letter to Terry and Jo Harvey Allen, 9/17/81

Biographical Sketch

The following notes are based on comments made by H.C. Westermann over a period of many years, as well as remarks and notes by his sister, Martha Westermann Renner and are intended only as a background for the letters selected in this book. Brief references to the USS Enterprise and USS Franklin are supported by information from the book *USS Enterprise (CV-6)* by Steve Ewing (1982).

I would like to make a general comment about one aspect of Cliff's sense of discipline and appreciation for independence and aloneness. Cliff's parents moved, after the birth of their first child La Nore, from St. Louis to Los Angeles where Cliff was born on December 11, 1922. They lived in a court built by his maternal grandfather, George Bloom. Cliff was always surrounded by family as most of the ten bungalows were inhabited by Bloom relatives. Later the Westermann family moved to a small two-bedroom house on Norwich Drive in West Hollywood. Cliff slept in the dining room and his closet was the hall closet. For the greater part of thirty years, including of course, military service, he had very little privacy or aloneness.

The impression Cliff gave of his father was that of a very quiet, private person. He was honest and hard-working and very neat in his habits and dress. His in-laws, with the exception of his father-in-law, disapproved of him and felt he was too unambitious and low-keyed. He lost his job as hotel accountant during the Depression, but was then hired by a firm with which he stayed until he died in 1963. The firm he worked for sent him to various hotels — Los Angeles, Long Beach, San Diego, Lake Arrow, and eventually Phoenix and Bakersfield. He was usually gone for weeks at a time. He disliked his name, Horace, and was referred to as either H.C. or Cliff, and was unhappy that his son had been named Horace also. His nickname at work was "Ace," which Cliff thought referred to his abilities as an accountant. However, one day after a trip to a pool hall he discovered the unexpected and apparently clandestine "Ace" in his father. Although they were not particularly close, Cliff always held his father in high esteem.

Cliff's mother, Florita Bloom, was the dominant figure, by necessity as well as by temperament. She and Cliff were very close and he always had great admiration for her. She was a talented and ambitious woman whose aspirations, including travel to exotic places like South America, were unfulfilled. The fact that she had to defer her ambitions contributed to Cliff's sympathy for women in general all his life.

It was his mother who started Cliff on a workout program because he was not strong as a child. She built him an apparatus in the backyard that was secured by guy wires and supported a climbing rope and a trapeze. She did the entire job herself. With her encouragement he became very strong and maintained a workout routine for the rest of his life.

Her aspiration for Cliff to become a naval officer was influenced by the career of an old beau who had become an admiral. To help his entry to the Naval Academy, she arranged for him to go to a military prep school by borrowing money from her sister Ruth Bloom. He had an appointment to the Naval Academy for June 1942. This later became a matter of contention between Ruth and Cliff. Florita had developed TB in the early thirties and as her illness grew worse her aspirations for Cliff became more intense. With the exception of Cliff's younger sister Martha with whom he always had a very compatible relationship, no one in his family was perceptive of his creative interests nor sympathetic to his nonconformism.

In the fall of 1941 Cliff left for military prep school. Just a few months later on December 7, 1941 Florita entered Olive View Sanatorium where she died in May of 1942. Cliff left school in January of 1942, unable to cope with the trauma of his mother's illness as well as the pressure of prep school and the entry of the United States in World War II. This was the beginning of his "being on the road," with its hardships and his meeting, in passing, many of the characters who exemplified the lost and the alienated and to whom he would refer in later years with empathy. He worked for the most part in logging camps and then signed up for the Marine Corps in Seattle in the spring. He was not heard from by his family until July of 1942 when his father received a letter from the Marine Corps asking for confirmation of Cliff's age and identity.

After basic training at Camp Pendleton, despite Cliff's wish to become a paratrooper, he was assigned to sea school and then stationed on the USS West Virginia for a short time. It had been severely damaged at Pearl Harbor and was being repaired at Bremerton, Washington. It was at Bremerton that Cliff saw the aircraft carrier, the USS Enterprise, arrive for repairs (after the Battle of Midway and Coral Sea). He fell in love with the ship and got himself relieved of duty aboard the West Virginia by, according to Cliff, deliberately failing inspection. He then volunteered for duty as a gunner aboard the Enterprise.

On March 19, 1945 a sister ship, the USS Franklin was attacked by a kamikaze just after the planes had been positioned on deck and refueled. There were huge columns of smoke from the ship, many detonations and over 900 casualties. Many men were trapped below deck. The Enterprise was ordered to escort the Franklin from the combat area. The next day the Enterprise was attacked. Cliff observed that dead bodies were carried to the stern and "stacked, nude like cordwood." From April 5th to 11th the Enterprise supported the Okinawa invasion until she was again struck by a kamikaze. The most devastating attack took place on May 14th when the forward elevator was blown 400 feet in the air by the explosion. In June the Enterprise returned to Bremerton for repairs after a stopover at Pearl Harbor where Cliff noted the smell of death from the Franklin that was still so hot that no one could board her.

A year later Cliff was discharged from the Marine Corps. He then went to work part-time for the Red Cross in Long Beach where he also spent a lot of time practicing handbalancing in the park. There he met Wayne Uttley who was also working out. They developed an act that was presented at the Strand Theater in Long

Beach and then taken on a U.S.O. tour for a year in the Orient. On tour he met and married June La Ford whose stage name was Penny Parker. Her father had been a comedian, and she and her sister Pepper had worked on the stage, dancing, as children.

In the fall of 1947 he settled in Chicago to attend the Art Institute where he studied advertising and design. His only son, Gregory Nat Westermann, was born August 19, 1948. During this first stay in Chicago he met Bruce Oxford who was to become a lifelong friend.

His marriage broke up in 1950 and he re-enlisted in the Marine Corps. He spent eighteen months in the infantry in Korea. His closest friend at this time was a fellow Marine, Paul Flowers who was nicknamed "Stick." According to Cliff, "Stick" was a quiet modest man who had been a professional gambler by trade. Cliff was very interested in his ability to win or lose with equanimity. He also sympathized with him because of his very remote relationship to his family. "Stick" died in Korea shortly after Cliff was discharged. Cliff's sister, Martha, had signed up for the WACS and was stationed in Japan and often sent Cliff packages of food. Although he rarely spoke of it, Cliff regarded his experience in the Korean War not only as difficult, but also as freeing him from the unwanted expectations of his family and the unhappiness of his failed marriage. The war in Korea made him question the role of the United States in that war and it also clarified his priority about becoming an artist.

He was ready to commit himself to being an artist and so returned (on the G.I. Bill) to the Art Institute in Chicago where he was able to study fine arts exclusively. He lived at 25 East Division Street where he spent several years renovating the building in return for room and board and in the process acquiring considerable woodworking skills. Cliff graduated from the Art Institute in 1954. He stopped painting and concentrated on making highly personalized constructions, the first of which was called *The City*. His first sale in 1955 was of a piece entitled *Butterfly* to Mies van der Rohe. In 1956 he met Allan Frumkin who would become his dealer and Dennis Adrian who worked for Allan Frumkin and would become a lifelong supporter.

I met Cliff through a friend, Irving Petlin, in June 1957, shortly after I had moved to Chicago from New Haven, Connecticut where I had been studying painting at Yale University Art School. I had seen the summer group show at Allan Frumkin's and met Cliff soon after. I was much impressed by him, as well as his "shop." I saw him at a few parties that summer, always alone, and immaculately dressed in a blue suit, white shirt, and black tie. We didn't really establish a close friendship until the winter and spring of 1958. My impression of him at that time was of someone very attractive, quiet and controlled. He was always polite and talked very little about himself. In fact, he talked very little. He seemed to have a leashed kind of energy and tension. There was nothing careless about his manner. He seemed to be very much apart, alone but not aloof. He never complained about anything. It wasn't until we got to know one another in the spring of 1958 that he showed his sense of humor or used any of the more provocative profanities with which he illuminated his speech. At first he would come over to my place two or three evenings a week and then every night and we would talk for hours and have a great time. Once I got to know Cliff I also knew that he was very trustworthy and loyal.

In the summer of 1958 I decided to get a divorce in Reno. I had been separated from my first husband in the spring of 1957 in Connecticut. On my return in September our friendship and love grew even stronger. Cliff had made some money from his first solo show with Frumkin and we used it to take a trip in February 1959 to the Yucatan. On March 31st we were married.

We lived first in a place on Dearborn where we took care of the building in exchange for free rent. We also did janitorial work for two other buildings in the neighborhood. Cliff had an excellent reputation for fine workmanship, modest estimates and reliability. Then we moved to 222 North Avenue to an old two-and-a-half-story building that Bruce Oxford had leased with his wife Doris with the idea of creating a coffee house on the ground floor. We worked there off and on. Our last winter in Chicago was very difficult. We had a fire in our building and we also didn't really have enough money. So after several invitations from my parents, Dorothy and Lester Beall, we decided to try living with them in Connecticut.

We ended up living with them from October 1961 to June of 1964. And it worked out well for us. We stayed in the main house but they gave us the cottage nearby to work in. My father, who was a graphic designer, had to go to New York several times a month and, since we did not have a car, Cliff would accompany him, with his work, to Frumkin's gallery. During this period we met Mike Nevelson, a sculptor who lived in a neighboring town, and the artist Robert Delford Brown and his wife, Rhett.

In the spring of 1964 we decided to take a long trip across the country and find a place to live out on the West Coast. Cliff bought a 1949 Chevrolet pick-up for $400. He spent weeks renovating it and building a small cabin over the truck bed. He made a lead casting of a bat-like figure for the hood ornament. We spent three months taking back roads all across the country, usually camping in a field or in the woods. Cliff would bury the trash each morning and on one occasion even swept away our tire tracks. In Jackson, Tennessee we stayed at a rooming house where we bought a collage done by a deceased elderly roomer which Cliff eventually gave to Walter Hopps. We also passed through Muskogee, Oklahoma where Cliff's mother had grown up and married. There we saw the house that Cliff's grandfather George Bloom had built. Each room was constructed of a different hardwood and the chandeliers were suspended from carved wooden chains.

We ended up in San Francisco by which time we had run out of money to do more exploring. We found a small apartment near Chinatown with one room for Cliff to work in and one for myself. Cliff made a number of pieces during that year from a very fine grade of Honduras mahogany that was readily available there. We met William Wiley that year at Peter Saul's studio. We worked out regularly at a very fine gym run by Walt Baptiste, a former professional Mr. America weight lifter and accomplished yogi, who became our closest friend there. But neither one of us was particularly taken with San Francisco. Cliff regarded San Francisco as a "city of insurance companies and alcoholics." He was fascinated, however, by the many news reports of suicide, usually via the Golden Gate or Bay Bridges. San Francisco had the highest rate of suicide in the country.

It was in San Francisco that Cliff felt that he had been successful for the first time in projecting the image of the Death Ship. He had made masts for this ship and numerous details which, after study, he removed one by one, leaving a form that was very spare. Then finally he cut the bottom at an angle, thus giving it a list. It was the list that he felt gave it its force of image. He used the naval term: "dead in the water." It was the first of many succeeding versions. It was a breakthrough.

Our return to Connecticut in October of 1965 was pretty impromptu and, I think, related to the logistics of getting work to the gallery in New York. Also, my parents invited us back. This time we lived in the cottage at a low rent. We remained there for the next sixteen years. That first summer Cliff's son, Greg Westermann who was then seventeen, visited us and stayed six weeks. Cliff had not seen him since a weekend visit to Florida in 1956. Greg wanted to join the Marine Corps. He had dropped out of school and had been working at a car wash in Florida, where he lived with his mother and her girlfriend.

From the time we had married, I had, at Cliff's instigation, worked out regularly and practiced handbalancing. Cliff gave me very good instruction and started me on rope-climbing and a headstand. He was a good teacher. Working out together was fun and almost a daily routine. In the fall of 1966 I joined a three-partner acrobatic act in Montreal called the "3 Renowns." But I was only able to return home two out of every ten days. Also I wanted to spend more time painting so I returned home in the winter of 1967. Unbeknownst to me Cliff had asked my father if he could build a studio that I could use. Cliff built the chimney, spending nearly three months on it from September to November of 1967.

I would like to note at this point Cliff's affection for animals. He fed the raccoons every evening — usually going to a day-old-bread place and picking up bread, cupcakes and sweets. Eventually he was feeding forty of them. He did this for a number of years until he was asked if he would feed his children such junk. From then on he fed them dog chow, after carefully reading the nutritional data on the back of the bags. Every morning during the winter, he would set out shavings of suet, gotten at the meat market, for the crows, and he religiously maintained a birdfeeder. The dog chow also attracted a rare fox or two. He continued this up to his death.

In the fall of 1968 Cliff was invited to do a suite of prints at Tamarind in Los Angeles which became *See America First*. This trip coincided with the installation and opening of a show of his work at the L.A. County Museum. During that time, he became acquainted with artists Ken Price, Billy Al Bengston, Ed Ruscha and Al Shean, as well as the collector Ed Janss.

Before my father's death in June 1969, my brother and I had each been given a parcel of land. Mine had my studio on it. We decided to settle in Brookfield

Center permanently, and build a studio for Cliff and a house for us that would be connected to Cliff's studio. This was only 800 feet from where we were living in the cottage. We started the task of clearing dense brush, as well as seventy-five adult trees, in the summer of 1969. This took us the entire summer as we had to cut and split the logs and burn the brush as we went along. The framing and roof of the house were done in 1970. But we would not return to work on the house section until 1979.

In the meantime, Cliff began to build his studio. He had been working all these years in the cottage where we were living. He started the studio in 1971 and then went on to start the breezeway and porch that would connect the studio with the house. The porch supports were made out of nearby hemlocks with the bark removed. The wide casing around the doorway from porch to breezeway was made from zebrawood and he carved the words "Zebrawood, Africa" across the top board. When we had the money, we would work on the building almost every summer.

In the fall of 1971 Cliff was a visiting artist at the San Francisco Art Institute and in 1973 he was a visiting artist at the University of Colorado. I went with him on that trip. On the way back we visited Ken and Hap Price in Taos, New Mexico and passed through Medicine Lodge, Kansas where Cliff's mother had been born. Among the friends that Cliff made in the early seventies was Herk Van Tongeren. Bill and Noma Copley had been friends from the sixties after they started collecting his work. Bill and his wife in the early seventies, Stella, bought a house near us in Connecticut. This was the time we met Ed and Sara Canright Flood through Dennis Adrian. Also we saw a lot of Richard Hollander who was a collector of Cliff's work. He bought a place nearby in Pine Plains, New York. And Cliff made several trips with Ed Janss and his family on his boat on the Sea of Cortez, Baja California. On the first of these he met Jim Corcoran who wanted to exhibit his work in Los Angeles.

Cliff was diagnosed as having hypertension in the fall of 1972 and put on a regime of medication which he would continue for the rest of his life. Then in January of 1974 Cliff was ill again and underwent three weeks of extensive testing at Columbia Presbyterian Hospital. He was seriously depressed much of this year because of the various medications and unable to work. Finally he recovered from this episode with new medication and a new doctor. He went to work for the first time in his new studio.

His health remained good until the early winter of 1978. By then his hypertension had worsened because of serious arteriosclerosis. He was admitted to New York Hospital and after being there two weeks he suffered a heart attack. His life was saved by a new drug not yet passed by the F.D.A. When I would arrive at the hospital in the morning he would be quietly sitting by the window absorbed in either letter writing or small watercolors. Although he always treated the doctors and nurses politely, institutions of any kind were an anathema to him. When his doctor would ask him how he was doing with his cigars, Cliff answered that he was doing just swell meaning, of course, that he was fully enjoying them. His last week at the hospital was spent trying to find a safe haven in which to smoke his one cigar of the day.

His health seemed to improve over the next three and a half years and with it his zest for work returned. In May 1978, his retrospective opened at the Whitney, organized by Barbara Haskell. This year also marked the end of his twenty year association with Allan Frumkin's gallery. In August of that year he established a new gallery association with Xavier Fourcade.

By 1979 Cliff returned to work on the house. A friend and artist, Roger Brouard, whom we had known since the early 1970s helped on the house for three weeks. During that time, I was visiting artist at the University of Colorado at Boulder. Afterwards, I took a short trip through west Texas and found the house in Marfa. I called Cliff to see if we could buy it. We both loved the Big Bend country and thought, we hoped, to go there summers to draw. Earlier in 1979 we had taken a trip to Abilene, Texas to visit Greg and his wife. Greg was stationed there in the Air Force after transferring from the Marines. He had spent two tours of duty in Vietnam during the sixties. After visiting Greg we took a driving trip down to San Antonio and across to the Big Bend country. We made a second trip in the fall of 1979, saw Greg, met Jo Harvey Allen, but unfortunately missed Terry Allen, and then we continued southwest to see the house in Marfa.

1980 was a productive year for Cliff. He continued work on the house again with Roger Brouard who stayed for seven weeks in the summer. We both looked forward to finishing the house we had begun in 1969. Also Cliff made a number of new pieces. He was very happy with his association with Fourcade and, in particular, with having more funds. He really enjoyed this year very much and his health seemed good. Cliff continued to work out on a regular, weekly basis as he had since childhood.

Early in 1981 the wire lath was installed in the house. The plastering was done by Gene Bowen and crew. It was a three-coat process and took them from April through June. Cliff was enthusiastic about their work. He made his last piece — *Jack of Diamonds* — with galvanized wire lath. Roger Brouard stayed with us for five weeks during the summer and helped put down the wide red-oak planks for the floor — wood that we had bought in 1970. We hoped to move in the fall. My mother, because of increasing financial problems, had put her house, including the cottage, on the market. We believed it was on the verge of being sold by September, with the closing in January, 1982. But before we could move into our house Cliff became ill again with what was diagnosed as early heart failure. He was given new medication and ordered to bed. He suffered a fatal heart attack on October 31st and died in the Danbury hospital November 3rd. It was the end of an incredibly wonderful and genuine man and artist.

—Joanna Beall Westermann

Text type Melior, Letter type Optima

Designed by Annabel Levitt

Produced by Fred M. Kleeberg Associates, Inc.

Jacket designed by Louise Fili from a watercolor of wood graining by Joanna Beall Westermann and an announcement by H.C. Westermann for his exhibition at the James Corcoran Gallery in 1974